Natural Pet

PRODUCTIONS

TAYLOR & BECKER

DR. BECKER'S
REAL FOOD
FOR HEALTHY
DOGS & CATS
SIMPLE HOMEMADE FOOD
FOURTH EDITION

BETH TAYLOR & KAREN SHAW BECKER, DVM

For all the animals who share our lives, and especially for Gemini and Tessa, the dogs who showed us that real food can save lives.

Thanks to all the animals and people who keep us learning.

Disclaimer: The information in this book does not take the place of medical advice or veterinary care.

You are in charge of nourishing your pet's body in a way that makes sense to you. Consult your holistic veterinarian for specific diet recommendations for the animals in your care.

ISBN: 9780982533123

Printed in the United States of America
Fourth Edition, First Printing, 2013

dog photographs by Tina Krumdick
cat photographs by Catherine Davis
book design by Rosie Harper

Very special thanks to Steve, Tina, Allison, Rob, Shawna, Mary, and all of our friends who edited, calculated, read and re-read this version to make it better.

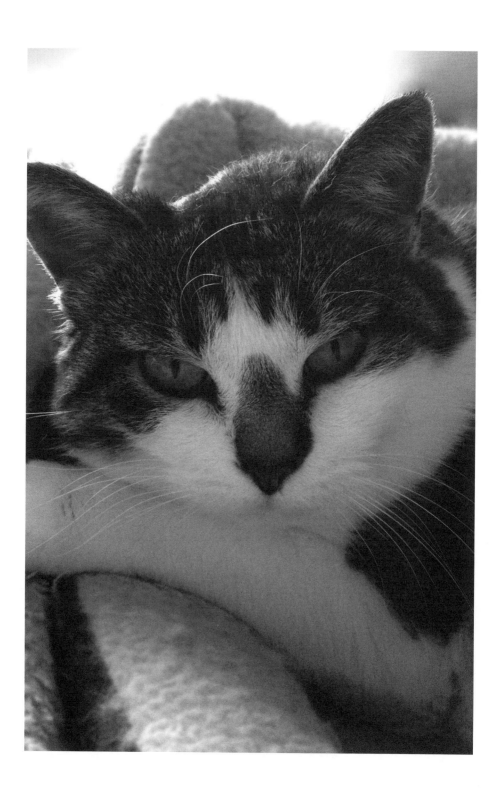

TABLE OF CONTENTS

Introduction 1

Chapter 1 – About this book 3

Chapter 2 – Food quality 11

Chapter 3 – The big pieces: protein, fat, carbohydrate and water 13

Chapter 4 – Additions: bone, minerals, vitamins, and fats 35

Chapter 5 – Preparation, equipment and storage 43

Chapter 6 – Recipes, feeding charts and transition 51

Veggie and fruit mix recipes for cats and dogs 55

Cats 59

Meat mix recipes – with bone meal added 60
Chicken with liver
Turkey with liver
Beef with heart and liver
Chicken with heart and liver
Turkey with heart and liver
Meat mix recipes – with ground bone 65
Chicken with ground bone, heart and liver
Turkey with ground bone, heart, and liver
Putting the pieces together 68
Rotation example
Proportions
Proportions for meat and veggie meals
Egg additions
About egg additions
Proportions for meals with egg additions
Sardine or salmon additions
About sardine and salmon additions
Proportions for meals with sardine/salmon additions

Essential additions
   Calcium
   Fatty acids
Feeding chart
Successful switching for cats

Dogs 90
   Meat mix recipes – with bone meal added 91
      Chicken with liver
      Turkey with liver
      Beef with heart and liver
      Chicken with heart and liver
      Turkey with heart and liver
   Meat mix recipes – with ground bone 96
      Chicken with ground bone, heart and liver
      Turkey with ground bone, heart, and liver
   Putting the pieces together 100
      Rotation example
      Proportions
         Proportions for meat and veggie meals
         Egg additions
            About egg additions
            Proportions for meals with egg additions
         Sardine or salmon additions
            About sardine and salmon additions
            Proportions for meals with sardine/salmon additions
      Essential additions
         Calcium
         Fatty acids
      Feeding chart
      Successful switching for dogs

Chapter 7 – Treats 123

Chapter 8 – Optimizing your pet's diet 125

Chapter 9 – A primer of commercial frozen products 133

Chapter 10 – Food for a lifetime 137

Appendix I – Mineral supplement 139

Appendix II – Analysis of individual diet versions 149

Appendix III – Bones for recreation or dental health 171

Appendix IV – Diet card 175

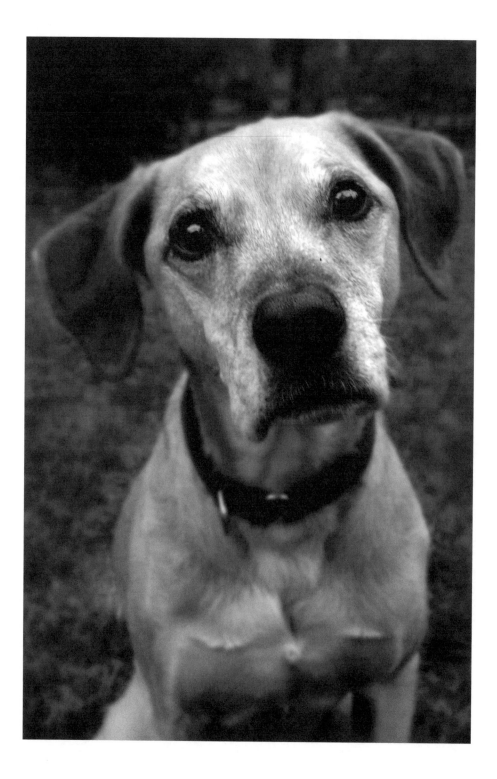

INTRODUCTION

We share our lives with animals because they're great companions. We want the same long and healthy lives for them that we want for ourselves. Good food, well-balanced relationships, clean air and water, plenty of exercise — these are the foundations of a healthy life.

We're told that humans need to eat whole, minimally processed fresh foods, and that we should vary our diets. We often get different advice for our animals.

"Experts" say never to change your animal's diet. Never feed him people food. "Feed your dog complete food in a bag." Most of us accepted this concept for many years — though we would look for another doctor if we got this advice from our pediatricians.

The truth is, food is just food. There's no "dog food," "people food," "cat food," "bird food" — it's all just food, with the balance and ingredients differing depending on the species. A fresh food diet is best for all living beings. A fresh, species-appropriate diet provides support for the body to maintain a vibrant state of being for many years.

Our advice: feed a fresh food diet. It's the most important component to promote a long and healthy life for your animals. You might see such radical changes that you'll be inspired to overhaul your own diet!

We need convenience in our busy lives. We want food fast, for our animals and for ourselves. The easy answer is dry food, the answer most of us accepted with little thought about the effect of dry food on general health. Food has not been considered very important for human health, let alone animal health. However, we are beginning to understand that there is no substitute for eating real food ourselves. The same is true for our animals. Many of the chronic and acute diseases suffered by humans and animals are directly related to diet.

If your dog or cat is already bursting with health, you may not see a big difference when you switch to fresh food. If she has chronic health problems, you are likely to see those improve. You may notice that some of the small problems you thought were "just age" have diminished.

We think you'll see and feel a big change.

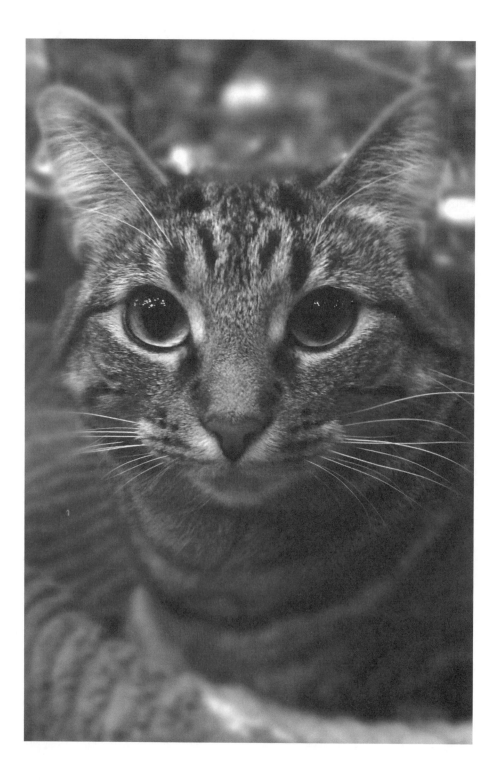

ABOUT THIS BOOK

Welcome to our newest edition! We've listened to the questions, suggestions and criticisms we received from all of you. We're grateful for the help, and we hope this revised and rearranged edition has been improved with your assistance. Though the plan is rearranged, it is very similar in composition.

Our goal is to provide a simple plan for a fresh food diet that supplies most nutrients in whole food form, using ingredients that are easy to find. Where there are shortfalls we give you ways to supply those nutrients.

We separated dogs and cats to make it easier for people to use the recipes and suggestions. This resulted in some repetition. In the previous edition we attempted to make feeding your animals really simple. It's still simple but we explained quite a bit more in many areas.

In the main text, there are lots of tables. You need to read these tables to find out how to put together the pieces of your pet's diet. Most of the time, once you find the information you need and enter it on a customized diet card for your animal (found in Appendix IV), you won't need to consult that table again.

Analyses of specific versions of our recipes are found in Appendix II. They provide you with details including protein and fat content, how many calories are in a pound of food, mineral and vitamin content, fatty acids and other useful information. We haven't included every possible variation, only the ones we thought would be either useful or interesting. There may be times when an animal may need to eat only turkey for a while, or has some other limitation. These analyses will help you to customize those programs.

This book is used by a wide variety of people, from those just getting into fresh food to veterinarians who need all the facts. If you're in the "new" category don't be intimidated. The day may come when you want to know all the information contained in those tables!

We want you to be able to see where you need to fill in the gaps in a fresh food diet, not just to take our word for it.

We revised the organ content of some recipes. We include the original recipe with same-species organs in the mix, but many people don't have easy access to specific organs like turkey heart, so we modified recipes to include more easily found ingredients (liver) and changed some meat components to maximize nutrients. We think it's better to provide the nutrients your pet needs in a form that doesn't quite equal a prey animal (chicken liver isn't found in a turkey) than to just leave out ingredients that are difficult to find.

Some mineral and vitamin supplementation is needed in a fresh food diet. Mineral supplement A for dogs or cats given in Appendix I covers the rotation given in this book. Use mineral supplement B if you are unable to include all recommended ingredients. If you use products other than those we describe, the serving size would change and you'd have to go through the whole process to figure out the serving size (complete with a gram scale), so we suggest you stick to the products we list. We prefer that you use our supplement or find one that includes the minerals and vitamins needed. You can certainly take the information given in the analysis appendix and formulate your own version.

To get the most out of this book, please read all the text before using the recipes, even if you've used previous versions. It's very tempting to just go to a recipe and start putting it together, but you need to understand the program before beginning. We've found that most of the answers to questions we received were to be found in the text people had not read. We hope that our revision, editing, and additions have made this book easier to use and read.

We can't include enough specifics to make the perfect page of directions for your particular animal, so we've added some "diet card" templates at the end of the book. Copy them and use them to write down each animal's diet program with amounts of meat mix, eggs, sardines, veggies etc. to make a meal, and include the amounts of bone meal, mineral supplement, fatty acids, vitamins and any other supplements you're using.

Periodically, review and make a new card. These records are valuable in tracing health history over time. Date cards when you start each one and you'll have a record of how you have modified each pet's personal diet program. On our website, naturalpetproductions.com you'll find that page reproduced as a PDF you can download and print.

There are lots of pages and sections here, but once you get going, it really is "simple food."

WHY MAKE YOUR OWN FOOD?

It's possible to buy commercial fresh frozen foods for your animals. Frozen raw pet food is one of the fastest growing segments of the pet food market. Some products are truly excellent, made by careful people who have given a lot of thought to the product. Others are poorly formulated with the same sort of ingredient manipulation seen in other pet food products (bony carcasses instead of muscle meat, higher fat ingredients instead of more appropriate lean ones).

Why would you want to make food yourself if you can buy good products? Making food for your pet is no small undertaking. Our culture is geared toward speed and convenience. The time it takes to prepare food can be considerable, but there are excellent reasons to make food for your pets.

- **You can save a lot of money.** Using the ingredients we specify and shopping carefully, your cost will be ⅓ to ½ what you would pay retail for similar frozen pet food products . If you use whole chickens and obtain a grinder, you can make chicken and veggie food for ¼ of the retail price. For turkey and beef, if you buy what's in season and watch meat sales, savings are similar. If your animal needs novel protein sources, the savings will not be as great, but you'll still pay less for your food.

  If you buy equipment to help you make food, you'll put out some money at first, of course. That equipment, however, will pay for itself over time and be useful for many years.

  Every time we make food, we can't resist figuring out how much it cost per pound and what we would have paid for it in a store. It's very satisfying.

- **You control the quality of ingredients and the recipe** when you make your own food. Pet food companies assert that they use top quality ingredients and claims of "organic" and "human-edible" may be true — or not. For example, when you see cantaloupe on a label, does this mean a lovely, ripe piece of cantaloupe, or does it mean rinds left from the preparation of pre-cut fresh grocery store products, or whole cantaloupe with rinds? Cantaloupe rinds can harbor molds, fungicides and pesticides. For the manufacturer, these options represent lower production costs. For you, it's not such a good deal. Fat is another concern. When you make your own food, you know the fat level. Labels give the percentage of fat as a minimum. It could be more, and there is often variation between batches. These are just two examples of many concerns.

- **Fresh food tastes better** and is more nutritious. Food you make is always fresher than food you buy already prepared. Several of our dogs, who leave commercial turkey food sitting in the bowl, became fans when we started to make it ourselves. Why? Was that commercial food "bad?" We don't think so. It just got a little old. It's still nutritionally balanced and ok to eat (though there is some nutrient loss in storage), but it doesn't taste as good. The long-term storage of commercial food affects nutrients enough that it's worth making your own food if you can find a way to fit it into your life.

You may be enthusiastic about preparing a fresh food diet for your pet. Or, you may be wondering how you're going to manage it. You might be convinced of the importance, but still worried about getting it "right."

This book provides a sound framework. As you become more experienced and knowledgeable you may want to add variations. If you keep to the basic principles presented here, you'll do well.

Our analysis of the ancestral diet comes from information gathered from anthropological studies and work done by Ellen Dierenfeld, PhD on the composition of prey animals (see the complete paper and other information at our website, naturalpetproductions.com).

Our food plan is designed to replicate the balance and content of the food dogs and cats really ate — mostly small prey, with some scavenging for dogs. The balance is approximately half poultry and half other meats and protein sources. You'll rotate through beef, turkey, and chicken, and add eggs and sardines to 8 of the 14 meals you feed in a week if you feed 2 meals a day. You'd revise this if you only feed once a day or more than twice.

A few individuals may not do well on the basic diet. Selection of the tiny and the giant in breeding, and breeding for certain cosmetic features or tempera-ment or working ability have left some of our animals with less than optimal health and function. Sometimes we see underlying problems that have been masked only when we switch to a more species appropriate diet.

For these individuals, a fresh diet is still possible, but it may need to be adapted to the needs of that individual. Some might need less protein than is included in this plan. Some might need more starch. Some might need more frequent feeding than the once or twice a day routine we're using here, especially tiny dogs. If you find that you're facing one of these challenges, work with an educated animal health care provider to adapt the diet to your pet's specific needs.

Our recipes may be fed raw or cooked lightly (except for the ones with ground bone). The issue of "raw vs. cooked" has been a major obstacle for many veterinarians and their clients in discussions about home made diets for pets. Is raw food safe? Is it appropriate for all animals? We think that food should be eaten in a state as close to fresh (uncooked) as it can be. However, there are many reasons why cooking may be appropriate or necessary. We think it is more important to eat a fresh diet than to be stuck in the fixed belief that food must be raw.

Use all the ingredients in the plan or your pet will be missing some essential nutrients.

This doesn't mean you can never vary your vegetables. It does mean you can't leave out the bone meal, the minerals, or the fatty acid supplements. You might look at your pet and say, "Oh, he's fine without that stuff, he looks great!" But, irreversible damage may show up down the road.

If you'd like to use our recipe with liver and heart, or the one with just liver, but you want to use goat as a protein source, you'll probably have a hard time finding goat heart. Of course we would prefer that proteins match, beef hearts for beef and chicken hearts for chicken, but if beef is all you can get, use it.

Skipping an important ingredient could have substantial effects on the health of your animal. For example, if you think you're following one of our recipes but the plan includes sardines and you leave them out, your pet's diet will be deficient in vitamin D and lower in fatty acids than is optimal. Without these nutrients, the immune system won't have the tools it needs to function and the critical balance of inflammatory chemicals (anti-inflammatory and pro-inflammatory, both needed) will not be maintained.

We find that the people feeding fresh food diets who drift the farthest from the balance of the ancestral diet are those who feed what is called "prey model." They are often feeding nothing but bony meats or chicken quarters. Because we feed only some parts of animals, other vital parts (spleen, pancreas, blood, brains, etc.) are missing. We need to make substitutions for the parts we are unable to find at the grocery store. This is done through adding fatty acids, minerals, and other nutrients. We are all for the "prey model" but this approach must include all the components that provide essential balance, and we just don't have some of them available – so we need to substitute, not omit.

Our veggie and fruit recipes specify certain foods. You'll see that we suggest in the text that you use what is in season, what looks good, and what's available within some guidelines. In this area, as long as you have variety, lots of color, and not too much fruit, the specifics can be varied.

Rotation is an important aspect of our plan. Over the course of a week, you will rotate through beef, chicken, and turkey, with eggs and sardines added to various meat meals. You'll supply your pets with almost all of their nutrients in whole food form.

We analyze our recipes as a complete program. Each recipe fits with the others. They are not designed to stand alone. You might be frustrated to find that there is not a "chicken recipe," but it's more nutritionally sound – and easier – to rotate through the components that comprise a diet with variety and balance.

If you combine a large meat mix recipe with the appropriate amount of veggie mix, the weight is less than 14 pounds. This amount will fit into most refrigerator freezers. If you make a batch of each meat mix and a few veggie mix choices, you might have a pretty full freezer but you'll also have good variety at hand. If your space is very limited, you could feed one major meat source recipe at a time and still provide good rotation.

If you find that you're leaving ingredients out and it's all too much trouble, you're better off with commercial frozen or canned products, or even dry food.

Really.

At least it's balanced and provides essential nutrients.

We're not all cut out to be full-time food preparers. If you've never spent lots of time in the kitchen don't let the first few batches frustrate you. It becomes easier as you get comfortable and find a process that works for you.

If you make food for a short time and decide that you're not inclined to "cook" for your animals, following this plan even for a while will give you great insight into commercial foods and you'll be a more educated consumer. Or you may decide that you're able to provide one meal a day of homemade food and the other meal will be commercial food. If you cook for your human family, these ideas are easy to incorporate into your routine. You may not cook at all for yourself now. After you make pet food for a while you might see the benefits and change your mind about food preparation!

Our recipes are in two sizes. Large recipes can be frozen in portion sizes that are right for your pet. The small beef and poultry recipes are enough for a day for a medium size dog, or more for smaller dogs and cats. These recipes may easily be multiplied.

If your dog needs a novel protein diet long term, with no ingredients he has been exposed to in the past, you will need to have that diet balanced professionally, because you won't be providing the proper minerals, vitamins and fats long term.

If you revise our plan for any reason and it becomes much heavier or lighter in any of its components, or if you subtract or add amounts, we cannot guarantee that the diet will be balanced or complete. This can be dangerous over time.

Whatever level of homemade food you can provide will be an improvement. Making food can be an enjoyable and rewarding part of life.

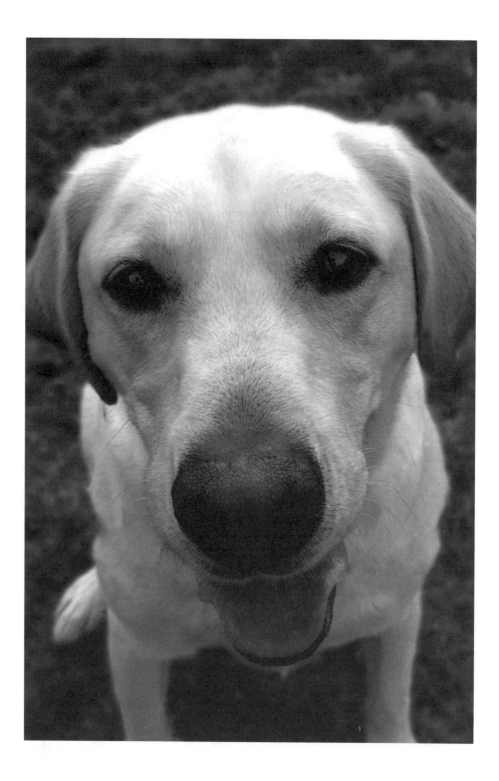

FOOD QUALITY

The meals you prepare with our plan will be superior to any commercial dry or canned food. Most dry and canned food is made from ingredients that are not "human-edible." Some of the reasons for this designation are relatively benign, but in many cases these ingredients have higher levels of various contaminants than is acceptable for humans, or even for food animals – animals that become our food. We don't think that our pets need these contaminants any more than we do. Some pet foods are made from better ingredients, but they are still highly processed and are stored for a long time. Frozen diets may be of good quality but most are kept in cold storage for long periods before they get to your animal's dinner bowl. Shipping of frozen foods is tricky and the quality of the food sometimes suffers. Any ingredients you buy will be fresh and significantly more nutritious than commercial food.

Many people choose not to make their own food because they can't do it at a pure enough level, so they feed their animal high-end dry food instead. Live, fresh food that includes the proper ingredients will always be easier to digest and assimilate than any highly processed food in a bag or can, no matter what the marketing material says. Fresh foods from the cheapest grocer are better than food in a bag. All foods found in grocery stores must be approved for human consumption, unlike the ingredients in most pet foods (even some of the best combine "human-edible" with "non-human-edible" ingredients).

"Natural pet food" companies – the ones that cater to those who know that a fresh food diet is best — use persuasive marketing to convince you that food in a bag or a box is just as good as real, raw food. People come to us and say "See? It's raw!" But unfortunately, after careful reading, we have to say "No, sorry. It's not." Raw food spoils and rots when you leave it out on the counter for a few days. Highly processed food does not.

Understanding the facts about what's true and what's not in pet food labeling and marketing involves a lot of research and learning. There are many resources available, but you still have to let that learning ferment in your brain until you can draw your own informed conclusions. You need some foundation information, and then you need to ask a lot of questions. This takes time. After you read a few hundred websites (from the conservative to the wildly speculative) and uncounted ingredient panels, we hope you come to the same conclusions we have — keep it simple.

Keeping it simple means feeding real food in a form as close as you can get to the farm or the garden. We probably can't raise our own animals and produce, but we can find the freshest and best available to our budgets and lives. If you can afford farm-raised and/or organic or natural food for your family, that's great. If you can't, you can still do very well.

We're for balance. We meet people who feed their animals at the very highest end of the food scale, while feeding themselves at the local fast food establishment. If you and your animals upgrade together to simply human-edible fresh food, with as little in the way of toxins as you can find in the supermarket, you'll be far ahead of where you started.

For very sick animals, quality is sometimes an even more important factor, because their detoxification processes are not working well. The lighter the load on the body, the better. If your cat or dog is ill, it's even more important to make sure you know every ingredient going into his mouth – and the simpler food is, the more likely it is that there are no artificial, toxic or highly processed foods involved.

There are many considerations in making this choice. No matter what you choose, you will be more critical of the quality of ingredients going into your companion's food than the most ethical of commercial food companies.

THE BIG PIECES: PROTEIN, FAT, CARBOHYDRATE AND WATER

In the ancestral diet of dogs, muscle, bone and organs make up 65% – 80% of the diet by volume. 90% – 95% of the ancestral diet of cats is muscle, bone and organs. The dry foods that most of our animals eat have a very different balance. The box below illustrates the radical change in diet that has taken place for dogs and cats from the diet their bodies were meant to thrive on. Looking at the calories provided by protein, fat and carbohydrate gives an accurate picture of diet composition.

The ancestral diet compared to dry food:
percentage of calories from each component

ANCESTRAL DIET	DRY FOOD
49% protein	25% protein
44% fat	32% fat
6% carbohydrate	43% carbohydrate

ANCESTRAL DIET	DRY FOOD
70% water	at most, 10% water

*the calorie % is determined on a DM basis

The balance of ingredients in our program by volume for dogs is 75% meat, organs and bone, and 25% veggies and fruit. For cats, the balance is about 88% meat, organs and bone, and 12% veggies by volume. This volume is slightly different from the ancestral balance. Although the vegetables and fruits take up a little more physical space than in the ancestral diet, the nutrition profile is very similar. In our experience, this balance works for most pets. The extra fiber from veggies helps out the intestinal function of our sedentary pets and the high antioxidant levels found in vegetables and fruits are beneficial for detoxification processes, rebuilding and healing. Some animals do better with a little less or more in the way of veggies.

Some medical or hereditary conditions require dietary modification. This program is for healthy, normal dogs and cats.

All animals are not metabolically normal. At the very tiny and the very large end of the spectrum in the dog world, differences in metabolism are common. In theory, *Canis Lupus* is *Canis Lupus*. Dogs are all identical in their DNA and therefore their physiology. However, in the last 200 years breeders have been quite creative. Many dogs and cats have been "line bred" or bred with their relatives to create or perpetuate specific desired traits, such as a certain color or size. This process can unintentionally result in the perpetuation of weak traits as well as strong ones, creating dogs or cats who may have weaker organ systems and in some cases have increased risks of birth defects and impaired ability to process and assimilate nutrients normally. Breeds that have been selected for specific behavior often also inadvertently carry negative tendencies. For example, many pointers have such a "wound up," high-strung temperament that they have a very hard time holding weight without some carbohydrate in their diet. This is just one of many examples.

We can still feed these animals fresh food diets, but the plan included in this book may not be completely appropriate. In the example above, the amount to feed would need to be increased to account for a higher metabolism, or additional carbohydrates added to the diet.

Cats, whose ancestral diet was primarily mice and other small rodents (moisture rich/high protein), have been bred and raised for many generations on "cat food." Their physiology has not evolved to process kibble, but their highly addictive taste buds have preferentially selected higher fat and salt foods. Cats raised on kibble who are offered their ancestral diet may not recognize it as food. Once cats are weaned onto raw food, they may do best with 90-92% meat and organs with less than 10% veggies (our 12% balance can be adjusted a bit). Cats and dogs suffering from kidney disease may require reduced protein levels in their diet. Work with an animal nutritionist who is qualified to help you modify the diet if this is the case with your cat.

Protein is the foundation of the diet of a carnivore, necessary for the formation of healthy cells, enzymes, hormones, ligaments, tendons, organs and protective tissue. Protein is an integral part of every cell of the body. Next to water, it makes up the majority of our pet's body weight.

The body can manufacture many of the building blocks to make the proteins it needs, but some proteins must be provided in the diet. These are the essential amino acids. Proteins help the body rebuild and repair. Organ and muscle meats provide necessary vitamins and minerals.

The bone portion of that large percentage of the diet contributed by muscle, bone and organ contains both the hard bone we see and the marrow inside the bone, which is mostly fat with some water, so "meat and bone and organs" really can't be thought of as just protein.

Fat in the ancestral diet comes from the fat we see when we look at meat, and also includes substantial amounts from bone marrow, eyes, and brains.

The fat content of the ancestral diet was higher in the fall than in the spring, but averaged about 6% of the diet by weight. Because fat has more than twice as many calories as protein, this 6% contributes about 45% of the calories (this calculation is done with the water in the diet first removed from the equation, on a dry matter basis).

6% fat by weight = about 45% of the calories

Though muscle meat, bone and organs make up a large percentage of the diet, when the ingredients are analyzed they look different. Because fat has more than twice as many calories as protein or carbohydrate, the fat adds up to almost half of the calories in the ancestral diet.

---

1 pound (2 cups) of 80% lean beef = 1129 calories

1 pound (2 cups) of 95% lean beef = 579 calories

If your dog eats 2 cups of food, this difference (allowing for the veggie component) could add 400 calories a day to our recipe, over 3800 calories a week.

In one week, this surplus could add almost a pound to your dog.

The diets of "raw" feeders who are not aware of this difference may be much higher than this level of fat, promoting an imbalance which may result in 75% of the calories (or more) coming from fat.

Fat provides fuel, essential vitamins and fatty acids. Fatty acids are necessary for a host of body functions including reproduction, normal cell membrane synthesis, normal healing and normal skin and coat. Dogs can get some of these fats from plant sources, but they do better with animal sources. Cats are obligate carnivores, and must get certain fatty acids (arachidonic acid) from meat sources. Fats are very delicate. At high temperatures or exposed to air, they spoil rapidly. Commercial foods usually include antioxidants to protect the fats, but fat still spoils quickly. Your fresh homemade food, with lots of variety, will give your animal more fresh nutritious fats than any commercial food.

The fat level of our program is at the level of the ancestral diet (about 6% of the diet is fat – which contributes more than 40% of the calories). Most of the fat comes from the food, with the addition of some fatty acids. The fatty acid additions are not large because most nutrients are included in their natural form – food.

More important information on fats can be found in *See Spot Live Longer*, available at our website, naturalpetproductions.com, and in Steve Brown's book, *Unlocking the Canine Ancestral Diet*, available from seespotlivelonger.com.

Carbohydrate in the diet of dogs comes from the intestinal contents of small prey and from grazing and scavenging. Cats also get carbohydrates from the intestinal contents of prey and they graze on grasses. In both species, small prey are eaten whole. With large prey or carrion, dogs often omit the stomach and stomach contents. For dogs, the carbohydrate portion might be as high as 25% or as low as 10%. Cats might average between 5% and 7% (these estimates are by volume, not on a DM basis). The calorie contribution of dietary carbohydrates is very low, but the vitamin, antioxidant, phytonutrient and fiber value is very high. We supply those carbohydrates with vitamin- and mineral-rich vegetables and fruits.

We use a slightly higher volume of carbohydrate than that of the ancestral diet in the form of vegetables and fruits to compensate for the sedentary lifestyle of our pets and to provide additional antioxidants to help the body deal with the inevitable toxins our pets encounter.

A review of wild canid and felid feces over a 30-year period confirms that the natural diet of these species does not include the high-carbohydrate end of the plant spectrum, grains and seeds, unless they are pre-digested by small prey animals (See our website, naturalpetproductions.com for the complete article).

Dogs and cats (and many people) are not designed to cope with large quantities of grains without long-term metabolic consequences, chronic illness and dysfunction, specifically unregulated inflammation.

You will not find rice, barley, oats or any high-carbohydrate foods in our program (except for small amounts of sweet potatoes and squash). For most animals, these foods contribute to poor gut health, slower healing, and the chronic inflammation that leads to general ill health.

We've worked with pets with skin problems, "allergy" issues, organ dysfunction, maldigestion, Irritable Bowel Syndrome, Leaky Gut Syndrome, and the entire array of immune system disorders that are influenced by diet. The healing of all these conditions is based in healing the gut. For proper flora to grow in the gut, so that all systems can work at their best, we need to put the proper food in that gut. Supplements can help healing, as can various modalities. But choosing to use foods that contribute to an unhealthy balance of flora in the gut is putting a large obstacle on the road to a healthy pet.

A starchy diet is a pro-inflammatory diet. The ways in which canine and feline bodies handle starches promote the production of pro-inflammatory hormones (certain prostaglandins and cytokines). Carbohydrates, in the form of grains, break down in the body to sugar. Carbohydrates require the pancreas to secrete larger amounts of amylase, the enzyme necessary to process carbohydrates, and insulin, the hormone necessary to balance the elevated blood sugar resulting from the metabolism of the grains. The drop in blood sugar resulting from the release of insulin signals the adrenal glands to secrete cortisol, a hormone that affects the body in many ways, increasing blood sugar levels and decreasing immune function. Over time, the endocrine and immune systems become stressed and off balance, leading to a host of degenerative diseases. These include immune system over-reactions (auto-immune diseases), immune system failure (chronic infections and cancer) and endocrine imbalances: hypo-and hyperthyroidism, adrenal over- and under-production of cortisol (Cushing's and Addison's disease and pancreatic disease (pancreatitis and diabetes).

When you look at your healthy dog or cat it can be tempting to say "He's really healthy, he can handle it." But what about if or when he can't handle it any more? Then it's too late, a problem has been created and you have no idea what other problems you've contributed to down the road. Keeping a healthy balance between pro- and anti-inflammatory hormones is a critical factor in maintaining health. It's better to be pro-active and maintain health than to try to remedy problems later.

Starchy foods like grains and seeds could definitely reduce the cost of a fresh food diet, and some feel this is reason enough to add them to the diets of healthy dogs and cats. When we look at our healthy dogs and cats, we aren't willing to make the potential health tradeoff. If you do make that choice, be sure you use a program that has been analyzed to contain all the necessary components. Most we have seen do not.

If an animal is in organ failure or end-stage organ disease, unable to process protein well, then he may need to consume more starchy vegetables like sweet potatoes or pumpkin, or even rice. These dietary alterations should be supervised by a veterinarian who has experience with fresh food diets – and who has the software to ensure that a lower protein, starchy diet still provides all essential nutrients. Choose carefully. Whoever you choose to consult should be able to actually analyze your diet to ensure nutritional adequacy.

Water is a dietary component we give little thought to. If your water is clean and toxin free, you're very lucky. Much urban water has chlorine and fluoride and other substances that are not desirable. For yourself and your animals, we suggest taking a look at your water. At the very least, a water filter pitcher (like a Brita®) can take some of the toxins out. Some water purifiers take out the minerals — we want to leave the minerals in the water. Bottled water might be a good answer, but many bottled waters are without minerals and others are no better than tap water. The use of bottled water certainly contributes to our recycling problems. Do some research on this topic and you'll come up with a solution that will be appropriate for your life.

MEATS

Our plan is designed to include all the meats and vegetables we've given you in the recipes. The nutritional analysis on the complete rotation was done with half poultry and half other protein sources: mostly beef with substantial (and needed) quantities of eggs and sardines. This basic program provides good variety and balance.

We'll briefly discuss some meats other than those included in the recipes so you'll have some information we think is important. If you decide to use different meat, the minerals needed and the fat balance will change some-what. As long as you stick to lean meats, and the balance of our recipes, you should be close.

At the grocery store level, careful shopping can reduce the cost of meat. Discount stores like Costco® and Sam's Club® regularly offer chicken at very low prices. Grocery and warehouse chain stores offer meat specials like round steak for half the regular price. Turkeys are cheap around Thanks-giving. Produce markets and ethnic stores are good sources for reasonably priced meats and organs. Independent grocers are sometimes willing to meet the prices of big chains if you purchase in bulk. Get to know the meat people — they usually love to help and can't believe that you're really making dog and cat food. They can tell you when sales are coming up or help you find exactly what you need. The trick for taking advantage of many promotions is storage. You must have room to store large quantities of food.

The meat we buy at grocery stores usually comes from animals that have been raised on antibiotics and fed pesticide-laden feed that's inappropriate for their bodies. It's likely that there are some residues in the meat that do not promote health. However, a fresh diet from grocery store ingredients is many steps above highly processed pet food in a bag or a can that's made from conventional grocery or lower quality ingredients. Even those products at the very highest end of the spectrum of dry and canned pet foods are still highly processed.

In "organic" or "natural" meat purchasing, there are no bargains. One reason to buy organic is that currently it's a relatively easy way to reduce the possibility that you are feeding meat (and produce) from animals that have been fed genetically modified organisms. There is much to learn in order to get what you think you're getting. It's beyond the scope of this book to educate you about this big area, but as with any product, let the buyer be educated. For example, "grass-fed beef" is trendy and it's better for you in a lot of ways than regular grocery store meat — but "grass-fed" may not mean "grass-finished." That beef you're paying a lot for may have been "finished" in a feedlot on grain, which means that the fatty acid balance you hope to obtain will not be present. This is just one small example. The best way to know what you're buying is to get your meat from small family farms that are concerned with good farming practices and the humane raising of food animals.

Resources abound. Natural food buying clubs and co-ops are not hard to find. Sustainable farmers have websites. When you start looking you'll be amazed. If you are limited to grocery store meats you can easily improve the fat profile with the additions found in the "Optimizing" section.

Remember that fat contains more than twice the calories as does an equal amount of protein. Our plan calls for very lean meats to allow space for good fats — sardines, krill oil and others. If supplemental fats (krill oil or other beneficial fats) are added to an already high-fat diet, the resulting caloric balance may be higher in fat than any other nutrient. It is very tempting to buy the cheaper, higher fat products like 75% lean beef. Often it's not imme-diately clear that the frozen "chub" of turkey is really cheap because it is 75% lean (25% fat) versus 93% lean like the more expensive product next to it in the freezer case.

You may read about dogs who are healthy on a diet that is mostly fat. This might be acceptable if other nutrition needs are met, but the conditions that make this work are not often found in the life of a pet dog, and never in the life of a pet cat – this would be a life in which thousands more calories were expended in a week than is possible for our pets. Working sled dogs, hunting dogs working in the field, swimming in icy water – these are situa-tions when a very high fat diet would be appropriate, when those calories would be burned for energy.

If a very high fat diet is fed under normal conditions, there will be less room for protein in an animal's caloric allowance. If meat is higher in fat than suggested, mineral levels and other nutrients will be reduced and the natural balance of nutrients will be compromised. If your animal's liver or digestive system is overtaxed, serious problems may occur and you may see a worsening of symptoms you are trying to improve.

We specify mostly dark meat of chicken and turkey in our recipes. Dark meat provides higher levels of some nutrients. You can use lean ground meats, too, if you desire. The discussion below is to give you a wider base of information.

Buy lean meat. The fat level of the natural diet of dogs and cats varies seasonally, but it averages around 7% of the diet as fed. Fatty beef, pork and chicken contain much more fat than the natural diet. 90-93% lean meat is what's needed to provide the optimal fat profiles found in our recipes. Check the fat content. Don't assume that you know. Turkey and beef are often 70% lean, 30% fat. Ground chicken may be high in fat. We found several "organic" ground chicken and turkey products that were very high in fat – but it took some label reading (and sometimes magnifying glasses) to figure this out. Organic or natural frozen ground meats are often made more affordable by adding fat.

People who make cooked food sometimes think that it is economical to buy cheaper, fattier cuts and drain off the fat after cooking. It seems logical, but after you drain the fat you have….less meat. It's no bargain.

Whole pieces of meat are easier to evaluate than ground meat because you can see the fat.

Does it seem that we are repeating ourselves about fat? We are. It's confusing that fat should have so many more calories than protein and carbohydrate, and it takes thinking about it a few times to get that idea integrated.

If you buy meat ground, it's safest to buy frozen "chubs." They have been frozen since they were packed, unlike "fresh" ground meat, which may have had inconsistent handling at the grocery store, increasing the possibility of a high bacterial load. If your grocer will grind meat at the time of purchase, this is less of an issue. Some ground meats have been subjected to various pasteurization processes. These products are usually free of pathogens but have they been affected otherwise? Opinions are mixed. They are, however, free of pathogenic organisms.

If you are cooking, inconsistent handling is not as much of an issue. Any heavy load of pathogens will be destroyed (though their byproducts may not, and this can be a problem). Buy meat that's fresh and not close to its "sell by" date.

Turkey thigh and breast are both easily found. In freezer cases, you'll find one- or two-pound "chubs" at reasonable prices, already ground. It's usually lean, but check. Sometimes the cheap products are 25% fat, a level that is too high for our use. Whole turkeys can be affordable, especially after holidays. You'll see organic turkeys in regular grocery stores and turkey farmers can be found not too far from big cities. For example, close to us there is a turkey farm that sells legs, thighs and organs for the cost of cheap chicken. To make use of these bargains, you need a big grinder, as turkey bones are too big to feed whole without some risks. You can debone a turkey, but it's a lot of work, and legs are impossible to debone efficiently. We've chosen turkey thighs for our recipes but you can use ground meat if it is 90 – 93% lean.

Chicken is a cheap meat to feed your animals, but don't rely on it for the entire diet. Variety is necessary.

Dark meat of chicken may have lots of fat you'll need to remove. Chicken breast without skin is lean. You may find chicken in chubs like turkey, but make sure to check the fat content — it varies a lot. Our recipes call for mostly boneless thighs. You can use ground meat if it is 90 – 93% lean, sometimes labeled 7%.

If you use whole chickens, strip the fat and most of the skin before using. Strip the fat from pieces as well. The smaller the chicken, the less fat it will have. Even organic chickens often have a hefty layer of fat under their skin.

If you cook your food, you can braise or stew a whole cut up turkey or several chickens in water to barely cover the pieces and then easily debone the carcass. Include the cartilage bits that attach at the ends of bones. Discard most of the skin and the bones. In the cooking process, most of the fat cooks out into the broth, so cooked poultry is quite lean. For storage, pack these cut up meats tightly in containers and fill in the spaces with de-fatted broth (chill the broth – the fat rises and solidifies). Poultry (chicken, turkey, duck, etc.) usually comes with organs and a neck. Cook these along with the rest of the bird, but pick the meat off the neck (cooked bones are too brittle to feed to your pets) and discard the bone. Chop the organs and add them, too. The amounts that come with a bird are not enough to satisfy the level of liver and/or heart needed – add organs as in the recipe.

Beef should be at least 90% lean. Our recipe is calculated using 93% lean. That's round steak or rump roast and other lean cuts. The names of beef cuts change in different parts of the country, so you have to educate your eyes and become familiar with the names. Look for meat with very little visible fat in the muscle (almost no "marbling") and remove exterior fat. Other cuts may be appropriate, but remove visible fat even from round steak if it has not been well trimmed. "USDA Select" grade meat is leaner and cheaper than "USDA Choice." There is not as much "Choice" meat in the display cases as in past years and for your pet's diet, that's a good thing. If you buy beef ground, the label will probably say "90 – 93%" lean beef. "Round steak" and "london broil" specials usually have quite a bit of fat on the edges. When we have had these specials ground by the meat department this fat was included, and the resulting meat was much fattier than the meat we trimmed and ground ourselves. There's no way to know the percentage for the home user, but we decided that we'd rather deal with it ourselves and be able to trim off the extra fat. You might find an enthusiastic butcher who is happy to trim meat for you.

Eggs (high omega-3) are a low-cost way to include beneficial fatty acids and excellent protein. The diet of the chicken is the key to the superior fatty acid profiles in omega-3 eggs. For high omega-3 eggs, chickens are fed flax. Chickens are able to convert the oils in flax into more usable forms of fatty acids (better than dogs and cats can). For high DHA eggs, chickens are fed flax and algae, with the same good results. Better food, better chickens, better eggs. This is an excellent example of the benefits of real food. High omega-3 eggs, like Eggland's Best®, have good fatty acid profiles and good levels of vitamin E.

Many "high omega-3" eggs found in large grocery stores come from sources that are similar to the regular ones – factory farms. The lives of these chickens are not necessarily better than those of the hens that lay the eggs that don't have good levels of omega-3 fatty acids. We can't all afford to buy eggs from hens that live natural lives, and these omega-3 eggs are a significant step up nutritionally.

If you can buy eggs locally this is always a good choice. Those chickens have spent some time in the real world, outside, and are likely to have eaten some real green food. The eggs from local chickens have better nutrient content than factory farmed eggs. They are an excellent choice for the whole family.

We include the equivalent of an egg meal a week (assuming you feed your pets twice a day) spread out over the week by including it with other meals.

You may cook eggs lightly, but keep the yolks intact and uncooked, to protect the fragile fatty acids from exposure to air and heat.

The "large" eggs we use weigh 1.5 – 2 ounces. The recipes are written as either "2 eggs" or in ounces "4 oz." If using ounces, you can be very precise, but in the versions that specify just a certain number of eggs, we have rounded them up or down.

Quite a few animals we know digest cooked eggs better than raw ones. In the evolutionary view, this doesn't make much sense, but it's not uncommon.

Fish is tricky. Our program includes sardines and salmon. We're warned against eating much fish due to heavy metal contamination and there are many problems with farmed fish. Yet, fish is needed in the diet for variety, fatty acids and vitamin D. Most of the vitamin D in our program comes from the fish additions. Only salmon and sardines contain significant amounts of vitamin D.

Canned fish is our choice. Canned sardines are small fish that don't live long enough to collect dangerous levels of heavy metals in their bodies. Sardines are wild, so the issues of what farmed fish eat and where they are grown are avoided. Buy sardines packed in water. Canned wild salmon is available in several varieties – just make sure it is wild caught. The bones in canned sardines and salmon are soft, unlike fresh fish. We've never had a problem with the bone aspect of canned sardines or salmon.

Much of the fish available to us has been farmed. Farmed fish don't eat their natural diet or live a natural life — you may be including some of the toxins you're trying to avoid. Genetically modified ingredients are probably in the diet of farmed fish. Currently (2013), it seems likely that genetically modified salmon will be approved by the FDA. We recommend making sure that all your ingredients are GMO free. Wild-caught fish are safest.

If you feed fresh salmon, cook it.

Some salmon carry a parasite (*Nanophyetus salmincola*). That parasite carries a bacterium (*Neorickettsia helminthoeca*) that is fatal to dogs who don't get immediate care. Freezing kills the parasite, but bacteria often survive freezing, and it is the bacteria that's the problem. This parasite is mostly limited to salmon from Pacific waters, but you can't be sure. The parasite has been found in other locations, and in other fish. It's easy to eliminate the possibility by cooking the fish. The fresh (cooked) salmon you feed your pet should be wild, so that it provides the best fatty acids and the best vitamin D level.

Bones in canned fish are soft, but bones in fish you cook at home are not. Remove the bones before feeding home-cooked fish.

Fish other than sardines and salmon might not have the nutrients needed for your rotation. A snack of your tuna steak will do no harm to the balance of the diet, but regular meals of fish other than what's included here would require nutritional rebalancing.

Below is information about meats not included in our analysis. To use lamb, rabbit, venison, and other meats, use Mineral Mix recipe B.

Lamb usually has a high level of fat. Many pets don't do well on lamb. Don't feel compelled to spend a lot of money on something that may be too fatty anyway. Small amounts of lamb may be included in the rotation for any healthy dog or cat. If you find a source of lean, homegrown lamb, use it!

Rabbit is usually available in ethnic grocery stores — it has almost certainly been frozen but check with the retailer to be sure. Never feed rabbit that has not been frozen. It is possible that very serious parasites may be present in rabbit that has not been frozen, but freezing kills the parasite.

Some rabbit specialty companies sell their products frozen or fresh. Fresh rabbit sounds like a great idea, except for the possibility of parasites. Buy rabbit frozen or freeze at 0° or colder for 72 hours before using.

Venison is a great choice for variety. If you know hunters, they are often happy to share, particularly organ meats. Since deer aren't raised with the same mass-production methods as grocery store meats, they probably have lower levels of toxins. We use deer organ meats, when we can get them, to upgrade the quality of a beef mix. If you can get meat and organs, that's even better! Do not use brains or spinal cords from deer. Freeze at 0° or colder for 72 hours before using.

Pork is reasonably priced and can be a good choice for a novel protein diet. Few commercial foods contain pork, thus most dogs and cats have not been exposed to pork. Keep it as lean as if it were beef (93%). Different cuts of pork vary hugely in fat content, and if you increase fat much in this program, you will upset the balance of minerals. Freeze pork at 0° or colder for 3 weeks before using.

Other choices include bison, ostrich, emu, goat, beaver, quail, pheasant, duck and other exotics. Explore these possibilities if you like but don't feel that you must. Pheasant has very brittle bones and should be well ground, not fed whole, to prevent possible risks. You can get enough variety in what's easily found to do an excellent job.

Organ meats provide high levels of minerals and vitamins. Ideally, heart and liver are important inclusions in a fresh food diet.

In the years we've been sharing food information with people it's become clear that some people who want to feed a homemade diet find it difficult to include organs. For those who can't find specific organs, we're including different choices in this edition. We can appreciate the difficulty of finding parts like turkey liver. We've adapted the "with organ" recipes to include only the organs we know you can find easily. The original recipes are still included.

In some poultry recipes for this edition, we've used chicken liver and gizzards in both the turkey and chicken recipes. This means you'll feed "chicken" every time you feed turkey and chicken. However, when you rotate through the recipes, the beef in the rotation gives enough variety that you won't be feeding chicken every day.

If you can't find chicken livers, beef liver and beef heart in your regular chain stores (some have liver only in the freezer section), look at your local ethnic grocer, where organs are abundant. These are the organs we include in recipes. Beef heart is easy to find and we really want you to include it. In the recipes with liver only, we don't include chicken heart or turkey liver because they're not easy to find. You'll find hearts mixed in with some brands of gizzards, which is great. Use them.

If you want to use heart and liver and they're difficult to find or deal with, you can get them from some commercial fresh pet food companies. You can add them to food or use them as treats. Manufacturers tell you how much freeze-dried heart or liver equals one pound of fresh meat. Check the resource page on our website (naturalpetproductions.com) for sources. These may be ordered direct or ordered through your local good-food pet store.

We include higher levels of heart and liver than would be in an actual animal to make up for the missing organs and blood that we don't feed. Thus a whole chicken would not have enough heart included to make up the amounts in those recipes.

The original recipes include organ meats from the same species. If you can't find them, you can include different organs. In a perfect world, there would be chicken heart with chicken. If you really can't find them, beef heart will do. In the case of exotic meats or even rabbit, you'd have a hard time finding liver and heart. So do the best you can. Just make sure you include organs. **If organ meats are not at the level described in recipes, use Mineral Mix recipe B.**

Tripe is often promoted as a source of beneficial enzymes and people pay a lot to include it in their food programs. Tripe is useful as a low fat protein source but unless you get it direct from the farm, enzymes have been washed away and often the tripe is bleached as well. Unless it's a bargain, it's not an important addition, and it's not a replacement for heart and liver. **Canned tripe is not a source of enzymes. Canning is a cooking process that deactivates enzymes.**

Gizzards from chicken are easy to find and sometimes very cheap. They're high in beneficial cartilage. Gizzards make up part of the "muscle" meat in our poultry recipes, but you can substitute an equal amount of muscle meat if you don't have gizzards. Some gizzards are packaged with heart – the label usually says "gizzards and hearts." There aren't often as many hearts as gizzards but some is better than none!

COOKED OR RAW MEAT?

Your carnivorous companion needs to eat a meat-based diet. If it can be raw, that would be best. We've seen thousands of dogs and cats recover their health on a well-balanced, raw, species appropriate diet.

We sometimes hear from people that their animal can't handle raw food. Usually this means we need to do some detective work. Often a problem that has been brewing is unmasked by the change in diet. Animals that don't transition easily are usually not in peak condition and it's best to pay close attention to the issues.

Sometimes the problem is the human who was under-informed about what comprises a fresh food diet, and we have seen some animals feeling pretty sick when their not-too-good digestion was expected to deal with two chicken leg quarters as a meal.

Some dogs don't like raw food or don't do well on raw food. That's ok. They may have reasons to dislike or have difficulty with raw food that you have not yet discovered. Their meat-based diet can be cooked. If your animal is ill, consult with your holistic veterinarian about the best way to start.

Animals who should eat cooked food include:
those who have had recent gastrointestinal surgery,
who are on chemotherapy,
or who have suppressed immune systems.

These pets should eat cooked food until they recover and have a good balance of normal flora in the gut.

Do what makes you comfortable, and what keeps your animal safe.

There are many ways to feed a fresh food diet. Start with the way that seems most appropriate for your animal. If you can't manage the idea of raw meat personally, don't let that stop you from providing a homemade meat-based diet. Just cook it. If you are repulsed by the idea of feeding your animal raw meat, don't do it. If you think that raw meat is dangerous, cook the food.

Do not cook bony meats!

Don't ever cook and feed whole bony meats (chicken necks, backs, wings, meaty bones). They become brittle and can harm your pet.

If you want to feed a cooked diet, use the boneless recipes and add a bone replacement supplement.

The tastes and needs of your dog or cat may change. Animals who have been happily devouring their food raw may one day refuse it. Some animals like their food warmer in the winter. Some prefer food cooked when they get older. In Traditional Chinese Medicine, there are conditions when cooked food is indicated and conditions when raw food is what's needed. These are just a few examples of when cooked food may be used, and it may be that cooked food is needed at some times and not at others.

Don't let your philosophy about food lead you to ignore what your animals tell you. Be observant and flexible. Does cooking food remove vital nutrients? Yes, but a well-balanced, cooked fresh food program is still better than your other options.

VEGETABLES AND FRUIT

What goes into your vegetable and fruit mix varies with the season. Choose what you include according to what's reasonably priced and available. Include as much variety as you can. Seasonal choices grown closer to home are fresher than, for example, an apple from New Zealand. There's no reason to include seven kinds of expensive organic greens (unless, of course, you're eating them, too!).

We provide some specific veggie mix recipes. In your day-to-day life, use representative veggies and fruits that are in good condition and in season as much as possible, locally grown when you can. There is a natural flow to produce available seasonally.

Grocery store produce has plenty of pesticide and fungicide residue. Pesticides and fungicide residues are hard for the body to get rid of and they are a serious burden to the liver and kidneys. Much of the pesticide residue can be washed off. You can use a wash product designed for the purpose, or you can use a very dilute solution of dish detergent with a thorough rinse — even a good rinse with plain water will remove much of the residue. Fungicides are used on potatoes, some fruits and winter squash. These chemicals are no better for you than pesticides and they're hard to get off. Unless you know your produce is free of fungicides, you're better off discarding the skin. The rinds of fruits like cantaloupe and honeydew are usually treated with fungicides, so discard the rinds. To be really careful, wash the fruit before cutting it open. Produce department staff can usually tell you how products have been treated. The boxes produce is packed in are often labeled with the preservatives used. Sometimes harmless wax is used, but it's still not part of a natural diet.

Do not assume that produce bought in health food stores is free of fungicides and pesticides. The same marketing goes on in those stores as in regular grocery stores, and sometimes it's even trickier as we become more susceptible to the "natural" designation. The more you know about the rules of labeling the better off you are.

Produce grown in the U.S. has been subjected to lower levels of pesticides than that grown in Mexico and other countries. California standards are about the best in the country in this regard. Grocery stores are beginning to post the country of origin of their produce as the demand for this information grows.

We have given you some suggestions on fruit and vegetable combinations, but we recommend rotating a variety of fresh produce, including asparagus, beet root and greens, broccoli, brussels sprouts,cabbage, carrot, cauliflower, celery, chard, chicory, collards, cucumbers, kohlrabi, eggplant, lettuce (all types except iceburg), mushrooms (medicinal mushrooms are excellent), cabbage, parsnips, parsley, peas of any type, peppers (not hot ones), rutabaga, spinach, squash/zucchini/pumpkin, sweet potatoes, tomatoes , turnips, watercress, yams, apple, apricot, bilberry, blackberry, blackcurrant, blueberry, cantaloupe, cherry, clementine, eggplant, fig, gooseberry, grapefruit, guava, honeydew, huckleberry, kiwi, kumquat, mango, nectarine, orange, peach, pear, pineapple, plum, pomegranate, raspberry, strawberry, tangerine, watermelon and any other pet friendly fresh produce you may have access to.

The more color the better — red peppers have more vitamin A than green ones, for example. Orange, dark green, red — lots of color indicates lots of nutrients.

Use mostly produce that is fairly low in calories. Keep the total of fruit and starchy vegetables (like sweet potatoes and carrots) to about 10 – 25% of the veggie mix overall. More than this amount will result in more sugar or carbohydrate than is natural for a dog or cat. We don't recommend corn, ever. Our program was analyzed with all the ingredients together. you may notice that some recipes are higher in fruit or starchy veggies: rest assured, overall the program is as you see it in the analysis pages in the appendix.

It's easy to make a big batch of veggie and fruit puree and freeze it. Because the produce is raw, it does not have a long freezer life. Those great enzymes are slowed down but not stopped by freezing. Make what you can use in a month or two and freeze in amounts you can use within a couple of days after thawing.

As you can see from these examples of starchy or sugary produce and those that are low in starch or sugar – it can be a big difference!

SOME STARCHY VEGETABLES AND FRUITS

	Calories in 1 cup	Carbohydrate grams in 1 cup
Acorn Squash	83	22
Apples	118	31
Bananas	200	57
Butternut Squash	82	22
Carrots	90	22
Peas	125	33
Potatoes	138	32
Pumpkin, canned	83	20
Sweet Potatoes	249	58

LOW STARCH/CARBOHYDRATE VEGETABLE AND FRUITS

	Calories in 1 cup	Carbohydrate grams in 1 cup
Broccoli	20	4
Celery	20	5
Chinese Cabbage	11	2
Greens	3	1
Zucchini	20	4

Note: the above figures taken from the USDA nutrition database.

Cut up washed veggies and fruit and puree them in a food processor, blender or Vitamix® — a little water can be added to make the process easier on the machine. Chopped isn't quite good enough – get your puree as smooth as you can to release all those great nutrients. The smaller the particle size is, the better the digestive absorption will be.

White potatoes have little to offer. The high carbohydrate level is not offset by high levels of desirable nutrients, as with sweet potatoes and winter squash.

Cook sweet potatoes, yams and winter squash for the best digestion. Always discard the peel unless you have grown them yourself, because potatoes and squash are treated with fungicides to prevent mold. Canned pumpkin is simple, but try to include fresh cooked sweet potatoes, pumpkin, and other squash, too.

Broccoli, celery and greens (which can include spinach, chard, collards, kale, endive, escarole, mustard, "mixed baby field greens" and others) are an easy veggie mix. Zucchini, peppers, cabbage, cucumber and parsley are another.

In winter, broccoli, greens, apple and carrot can be a good start. In summer there is much more variety at a reasonable price — use melons, tomatoes, zucchini and whatever looks good.

Plentiful fruits like apple, pear, orange, berries, tomatoes and melons of all kinds provide a wide range of nutrients. Papaya and pineapple are potent sources of the enzymes needed to help digest food, and berries of all sorts are intense blasts of antioxidants.

Don't feed foods in the broccoli family every day. This nutritious family, the brassicas, includes kale, cabbages of all sorts, collards, broccoli, cauliflower, broccoli-raab, bok choy and others. If you fed (or ate) these vegetables in very large amounts every day for an extended period they could cause a problem with iodine uptake, which might impact thyroid balance. Plan a couple of days a week with nothing in your veggie mix from the broccoli family.

A little more about the brassica family…some animals have significant gas and flatulence when they eat these foods. Fresh diet enthusiasts get very excited about all the wonderful nutrients in, for example, kale and collard greens. It's true that these foods are excellent sources of various minerals, but consider the results with your particular animals in making up your mix.

Try them yourself. The flavors can be strong and bitter. Milder greens can be just as nutritious. If you don't want to eat it, odds are your cat won't touch it.

Green beans and all other legumes are more digestible cooked than raw.

Health conscious humans often want to share their "healthy" foods (sprouted mung beans, lentils, brown rice) with their pets. If you feed legumes, sprouting and thorough cooking will make them easier to digest. However, including these higher starch ingredients in your pet's diet would change the nutrition balance of this program considerably. The result would be reduced levels of beneficial fats and necessary minerals. We don't find a place for the dry legumes (lentils, navy beans, etc.) in the ancestral diet of dogs and cats.

Frozen vegetables may be used. They're harvested at their peak and if they've been stored well, the nutrition content is good. Use frozen vegetables in conjunction or rotation with fresh. For those people in locations far from major population centers, where fresh veggies are sometimes limited in grocery stores in winter, frozen veggies can be an excellent standby.

Our veggie puree recipes are specific, but you can use the information above to vary them without changing the nutrient balance much. If you substitute, use similar colors and starch levels.

What should you leave out?

- Exclude onions, which cause Heinz body anemia in cats and dogs. Garlic is not metabolized the same way as onion. Small quantities of fresh garlic are fine for dogs and cats.

- Raisins (and grapes) may cause organ toxicity in some animals. Mycotoxins are a common contaminant of grapes and raisins. These toxins are harmful at very low levels. Read *See Spot Live Longer* for more on mycotoxins, one of the main contaminants of dry food.* It has not been proven that mycotoxins are the cause of the organ damage seen with raisins and grapes, but this issue alone is a good reason to avoid them.

* *The pervasive and dangerous nature of mycotoxins is a compelling reason to eliminate dry food from your pet's diet.*

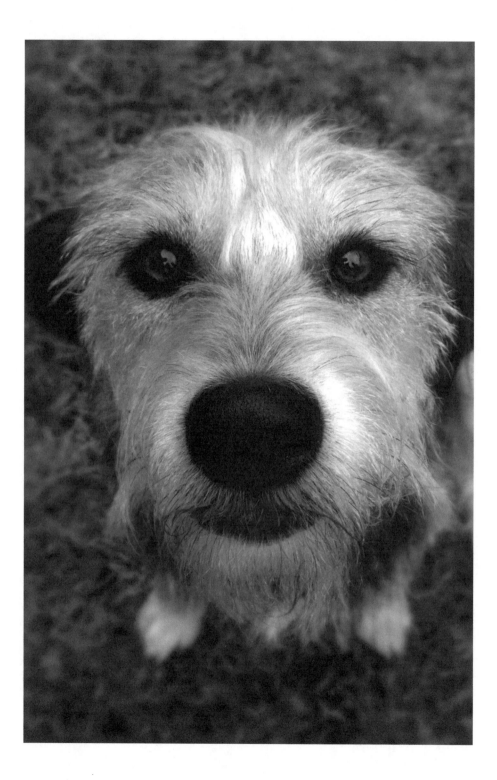

ADDITIONS

Your goal is to provide good fuel so that your pet's brilliantly designed body can do its job. Fresh food provides most of those ingredients, but some additions are needed to complete the diet. These include a bone replacement, fatty acids to balance the fats, salt and some minerals and vitamins that are in short supply in fresh foods for several reasons: the ways that we raise our food animals, the depletion of minerals from our soil, and the body parts (kidney, blood, etc.) that we are unable to supply.

Any homemade diet, however well balanced, will be short in some trace minerals. You could do it all with real food if you were willing to consider some odd and/or expensive ingredients. We don't want to make the process more complicated. Our goal is simple food. **You must supplement specific minerals and vitamins that are low in a homemade diet. The amounts are sometimes tiny but still essential for long term vitality.**

Consider that we humans eat many foods that are fortified. We don't even think about it. Vitamin products for humans are usually designed to provide 100% of most needs. Dietary deficits are much less likely for us. Commercial pet foods are designed to provide 100% of dietary needs, so pet supplements are for specific purposes or to add a little more of some nutrients, not usually to supply the entire daily requirement. Most pet supplements we looked at fall short, because they are designed as a "booster," or for a specific purpose. They may provide useful nutrients, but are lacking in proper minerals, even the ones that claim to be for homemade diets. You can use the tables provided in Appendix II to try to find a product that meets your needs. In our previous edition, we gave you a recipe to make a mineral/vitamin supplement to cover the shortfalls of a fresh food diet. In this edition, we added an appendix providing analysis of the complete diet program and some recipe versions in an appendix. In the charts you'll find the nutrients needed to make sure essentials are covered. In Appendix II, you'll find two examples of a homemade supplement for cats and two for dogs.

When buying supplements like bone meal, enzymes and fatty acid supplements, vary your products when you can. Find a couple of brands at least and rotate through them. Sometimes the acceptable choices are limited. In general, buy small quantities and try a different brand when you're ready to purchase again.

The quality of supplements varies – make sure you investigate the products you purchase.

REPLACING BONE IN THE DIET

"Bone" in supplement form is necessary for proper calcium and phosphorus balance in diets that use boneless meats. You'll find tables that give you the appropriate amounts to add based on the calcium content of the bone meal, and some examples using different products

If you feed recipes with bony meats (or any raw diet program with a balanced amount of calcium), do not add calcium or bone meal.

Calcium supplements that do not provide phosphorus are not appropriate. Calcium alone does not build the replica of the ancestral diet we're aiming for. Bone has substantial amounts of phosphorus and other minerals critical for building and maintaining a vibrant body.

The calcium comparison chart on the next page shows you how different the results are when a calcium-only product is used.

Without the balance of phosphorus and calcium contained by bone, the phosphorus would be very low, *and the calcium and phosphorus level and ratio would be inadequate for puppies or high fat diets.* Bone meal is the best way to mimic the balance of the ancestral diet.

The difference between meat with just calcium added and meat with bone meal added

Shaded boxes show where meat + only calcium does not meet minimum standard for growth. (We show dog requirements here for illustration purposes only.)

	AAFCO requirement for growth	meat only (no bone supplement)	meat + 2% egg shells	meat + 2% plant (coral) calcium	meat + 2% bone meal
calcium, grams per 1000 kcal	2.9 grams	0.1 grams	3.1 grams	2.7 grams	3.1 grams
phosphorus, grams per 1000 kcal	2.3 grams	0.6 grams	0.6 grams	0.7 grams	1.7 grams
calcium/ phosphorus ratio per 1000 kcal	1:1 to 2:1	0.17: 1	5.2: 1	3.9: 1	1.8: 1

Both "calcium only" additions, eggshells and plant (coral) calcium, put the calcium level higher than desired, and the phosphorus levels are not high enough for growth. The ratio of calcium to phosphorus is not acceptable with these products.

Bone meal is ground, cooked bone with the protein, fat and water removed. It provides the minerals of whole, raw bone without the fat, water and protein that come along with fresh, raw bone. Human edible bone meal made in USDA plants has a certificate that it has been tested for heavy metals and other contaminants. In order to be used by a USDA company, each batch of bone meal must have its own certificate that it passed this testing. Good pet supplement companies can sometimes document that heavy metal testing for their products has been done. **Do not use bone meal intended for the garden.**

When you calculate the amount of bone meal your pet needs, make sure you are looking at the amount of calcium, not the amount of bone meal. Include the amount of bone meal that contains enough calcium to meet your pet's needs. Bone meals range from 20 – 33% calcium (calcium being the easiest way to compute serving size). This can make a large difference in serving size, as much as ⅓ more or less. For our purposes, we've chosen to use products in the 24 – 30% range. The products listed are examples, and it's easiest to use one of those. If you don't use one of our suggestions, use the table that follows the Bone Meal Serving Size table to compute your serving size. Read all labels closely. Products change, and labels do not always make sense. Call the company if you can't find out how much calcium is in their product.

Dicalcium phosphate (available at some pet stores and online) may be used instead of bone meal if you prefer. Use the calcium tables for cats and dogs to find the amount needed.

Calcium citrate is a good choice *if there is a medical reason for your adult pet's diet to have restricted phosphorus.* If your pet does not have a medical condition requiring that phosphorus be restricted, use one of the other options. Do not use for growing puppies and kittens.

FATTY ACIDS

Fats are composed of many fatty acids: saturated fats, monounsaturated fats, and polyunsaturated fats. All these forms of fats are needed in the diet. Proper balance and amounts require some planning and knowledge of the nutrients involved. AAFCO only requires linoleic acid. We believe animals do better with a balanced fatty acid profile, so we have chosen to follow NRC recommendations for fats in our recipes.

We are mostly concerned with three main types of omega-3 fats:

- EPA (Eicosapentaenoic Acid)
- ALA (Alpha-Linolenic Acid)
- DHA (Docosahexaenoic Acid)

Most of the significant health benefits associated with omega-3 fats are linked to animal-based omega-3 fats like EPA and DHA. In some cases a diet may be deficient in a specific omega-6, linoleic acid (beef diets).

We've suggested using krill in our recipes because krill has some benefits not found in most fish oil. Krill oil contains eicosapentanoic acid (EPA) and docosahexanoic acid (DHA) in a phospholipid form. The unique phospho-lipid structure makes krill oil more absorbable and krill provides phosphatidylcholine, a natural source of choline, which particularly benefits the liver and brain. Additionally, there is an astaxanthin molecule attached to the EPA phospholipid. This potent antioxidant adds an extra benefit that most fish oils don't have (some salmon oils also contain astaxanthin).

We believe each oil has merits and benefits, and we recommend you rotate oils to provide all of these benefits to your animals.

Fatty acids are included in the food plan. The canned sardines and high quality eggs we recommend provide fatty acids as an integral part of their makeup. Krill oil or other oils are part of the plan, too. The recommended supplemental oil amounts are intended for those who are feeding our diet plan, which provides omega-3 fatty acids including DHA and EPA. With the sardines or salmon and eggs you'll be feeding, supplemental amounts of fatty acids needed are small. Adding more krill or fish oil wouldn't make up for excluding sardines and eggs. It is very easy to exceed the safe upper limit for fat when adding fatty acid supplements.

Fatty acid supplements don't keep well. Take them yourself, too, and they will be used quickly. There are no bargains in oil supplements. This is an area where cheap products may be more harmful than beneficial. Use only prod-ucts that can be proven to be free of heavy metal contamination. Products that have been tested are usually advertised this way. Testing information for each batch is often available on company websites. Pet product sales people may say that they have a great product, but before you buy, do some research. The same is true for human products.

Possibilities for other fatty acid supplements:

- Salmon oil
- Squid oil
- Anchovy oil
- Sardine oil

There are many choices. If you have small animals and you're using a liquid fatty acid supplement, buy small bottles. Small bottles are more expensive but if you buy large bottles you will be feeding rancid, spoiled oil before you get to the end. Glass bottles protect liquid contents best. Some products only come in capsules. Capsules keep the oils preserved the best but may be annoying to poke or snip to open for small pets. We give small animals a bit from a snipped capsule and take the rest ourselves – it's not precise but it works for us!

You'll find the recommended amounts of required fatty acid supplements with the calcium charts in the recipe chapter, with some information about the various products, and a table to help you calculate serving size.

In the "Optimizing" chapter, we suggest small amounts of plant-based oils to provide better ratios of LA (linoleic acid, an omega-6) and ALA (an omega-3) in our grocery store meats. *If you feed only beef for some reason, you must use hemp oil another supplemental oil that provides linoleic acid – without it your diet will be deficient in LA, an essential nutrient.*

FIBER

Fiber may be needed because we don't feed our animals fur and other non-digestible sources of fiber, or they may be constipated because they live sedentary lives. If your pet has dry, crumbly stools or difficulty defecating, add fiber. If your pet does not have dry crumbly stools or trouble defecating, do not use a fiber supplement unless recommended by your veterinarian.

Ground psyllium or coconut fiber (chips or flour) are both easy ways to add insoluble fiber if needed, but often more pumpkin or veggies will take care of a problem.

Dog's Weight	5#	10#	25#	40#	50#	75#	100#
Ground Psyllium or coconut fiber per meal	⅛ t	¼ t	½ t	¾ t	1 t	1¼ t	1½ t

Cats: ¼ t per cat should be sufficient

NON-ESSENTIAL but desirable daily additions to a basic diet include

- a glandular product
- digestive enzymes
- probiotics

We'll discuss those in the "Optimizing" chapter.

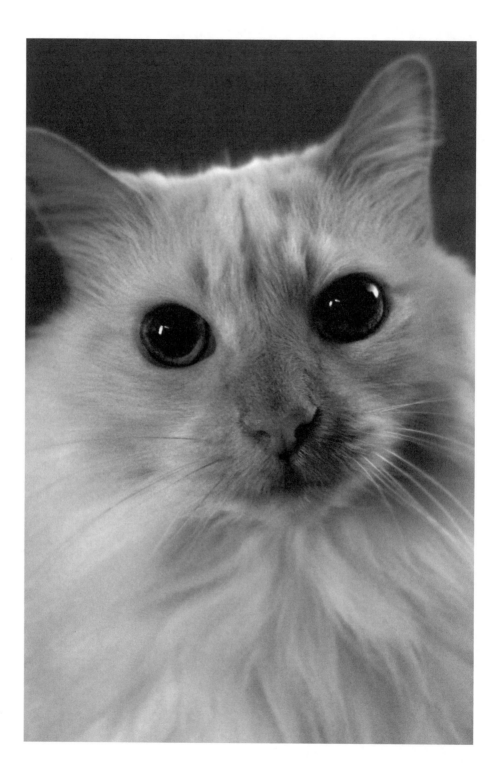

PREPARATION PRINCIPLES, EQUIPMENT AND STORAGE

Dogs are built to be able to digest carrion (dead animals) and all the bacteria (both good and bad) inside those animals, but their digestive systems aren't always in great shape. Both dogs and cats frequently suffer from poor digestion. Both pets and humans need to be protected from toxic food. Pathogens multiply rapidly at room temperature. Simple food preparation guidelines keep everyone safe. In cold weather it's easy to keep things cool while you make food, but in warmer weather pathogens grow more quickly as food warms up. The following guidelines will help keep your fresh meat safe and your produce from losing valuable phytonutrients and vitamins. Remember, you are using all "human" ingredients. There are no more bacteria on your cutting board after making "dog food" than there are after you prepare dinner for your family. Use the same common sense and disinfecting procedures for both.

PREPARATION

Prepare food quickly. Air and heat are enemies of nutrition. Meat needs to stay cold to keep pathogens from multiplying and to preserve the quality of the meat. Warm produce loses vitamins very rapidly. Once you have pureed your veggies they lose significant nutrition if not kept airtight and frozen quickly. If you're making food for a day or two, this is easy to do, but if you're making big quantities it's more of a challenge. Refrigerate the parts you're not working with. Keep things cold! Coolers can be a great help, with a bag of ice on the bottom. Make sure you're prepared before you start.

Food must be frozen quickly and it must be protected from air to preserve fragile nutrients. On food preparation days, get your freezer space organized so that you can spread out your containers for the fastest cooling/freezing. Stacking freezer containers tightly will result in very slow freezing. You may find unfrozen contents as much as two days later. Existing pathogens can multiply in these conditions. This is important for both meat and veggie mixes, as vitamins and phytonutrients are lost when exposed to air and light. Your freezer may have a "quick-freeze" setting — use it!

Keep utensils and containers clean. Processing meat (or even veggies) can be a messy process! If you're making a lot of food, clean up every hour or so. Wash everything with hot soapy water, and begin again. Scrub bowls, knives, counters and food processor containers. Use common sense. The food that you're putting in that giant bowl may be cold, but if the bowl is being used for the fifth time, leftover food on the edges could be quite warm.

STORAGE

Good storage is essential for food safety and palatability. It's distressing to put effort, time and love into making a great batch of food and have it spoil or lose quality from poor storage. Freezer-burned food has lost nutrition, and it tastes like old ice cream or frozen pizza that fell to the bottom of the freezer for a year.

Containers must keep food protected from air. The easier they are to wash and store, the better your food preparation experience will be. Freezing food in amounts that will be used in a day makes for fast thawing and easy rotation, but for some people (those with multiple animals especially) larger containers may work better.

Veggies and meat thaw in different ways. Packages that have just meat mix in them thaw steadily and don't exude a lot of juice, and you can use the meat mix as it thaws. Packages with veggies let go of their liquid as they thaw. That liquid is an important source of vitamins and other nutrients, so try to completely thaw the package and give it a stir before using the contents.

The ideal container for freezing is glass, which provides the best protection from air. Freezer jars have straight sides and are made from glass designed to withstand repeated freezing. These jars, which can be reused indefinitely, waste no resources and impart no plastic substances to the food. Disadvantages are that they take up a lot of storage space and are very expensive. Sizes are limited. With glass, defrosting takes more thought – you don't have the option of immersing containers in cool water because the change of temperature can cause them to crack. Over time, glass containers pay for themselves — they don't wear out. For families with lots of animals or big animals, glass is not easy to use, but if you are committed to the best possible storage this is your choice.

It is tempting to use recycled glass for freezing and many times it works pretty well, but most recycled glass containers were not designed to stand up to freezing and a significant number of them will crack with repeated use. Straight sides are needed: the expansion of contents can break glass jars at the shoulder. Even using appropriate shapes of recycled glass containers, more breakage will occur from the expansion of contents than if freezer jars are used. The result is food that must be discarded, so this is not necessarily a money-saving choice.

Plastic containers range from food industry grade (expensive, long wearing and relatively non-toxic) to semi-disposable. The quality of the food industry containers is excellent, but to buy enough for two medium size dogs for a month is a hefty purchase. They nest inside each other and take up less space than glass. You can find them at restaurant supply houses, online, and in stores specializing in cooking or storage supplies. Semi-disposable containers, designed to hold up through about five uses, are fairly durable and last far longer than five uses. They also stack well for storage and freezing and protect food well. When they start to crack, recycle them. Plastic containers of all kinds are available in many sizes.

If you're really thrifty and if using plastic is ok with you, other used plastic containers do a good job of protection and are often sturdier than the semi-disposable ones. Cottage cheese containers, ricotta and yogurt — many containers can be reused. If all your containers are the same, storage organization is easier, but free is good!

A number of the frozen food companies use excellent plastic containers and we really appreciate those! These 2- and 8-pound containers hold up to repeated uses. We love the foods that came in them too!

Home freezers are not as cold as commercial operations. Food doesn't cool as fast in home freezers. The bigger the container, the slower it freezes. A two-pound container freezes rapidly, but an 8-pound container might still be soft in the middle a day later. Pathogens can multiply and vitamins are lost in slow freezing. If you know how your freezer works and take this into consideration, you can use bigger containers safely. Spread them out and don't overload the freezer. There must be air space around containers as they freeze.

Plastic bags can be used, but they should be designed for the freezer. Regular bags don't do a good job of protecting food from air. Freezer bags aren't as easy to stack and store in the freezer as rigid containers and they're not easy to reuse. If you're storing food for a long time, even freezer bags should be double-bagged. You can store a batch of smaller bags inside one large bag and still get the protection of double bagging.

Label all containers. You may think that you will remember what you put in those containers and you may think that your abbreviation is perfectly clear, but trust us — it's best to label your containers clearly with enough words so that you really know what you meant. Currently there is a container in one of our freezers that reads "beefCa CK heart/liver tripe." What's in there is a mystery. It's wise to date containers while you're at it. Masking tape or freezer tape both work well. Label containers before you fill them. After they are filled, they will sweat – labels and marker will not adhere to the plastic.

EQUIPMENT

You can get by with almost no equipment starting out, but a few basics are needed or you'll have a big surprise trying to find a container to mix ten pounds of food.

A really big bowl is needed. Stainless steel is cheap and durable. Several very large bowls wouldn't be excessive. Plastic isn't the best choice for many reasons. Aside from the environmental reasons to avoid plastic as much as possible, most plastic bowls tend to hang on to grease. They become unpleasant to handle and hard to clean. The grease that hangs on becomes rancid — not something you want to add to your nice fresh food.

Real measuring spoons and cups help you to be accurate. Stainless steel is a good choice for measuring spoons, too. Dry measuring cups, which you fill and then level, give an accurate measurement for our purposes. Glass cups are easier to keep clean, but for semi-solid food it's hard to know exactly how much you have in a glass cup. Dry measuring cups are usually plastic or stainless steel.

Knives and cutting boards are pieces of equipment you may already have. Keep your knives sharp and use separate cutting boards for veggies and meat if you're doing both on the same day. The same sanitation requirements exist as for preparation of "human" food. A cutting board used for meat for several hours could develop some unpleasant inhabitants. Scrub and sanitize cutting boards after use.

Gloves may be useful. Hands get amazingly cold when you make a lot of food and after you wash your hands about twenty times they get a bit dry! Whether you choose disposable gloves or those that are more heavy duty, don't feel like a coward if gloves sound like a good idea to you.

A food scale will help you know exactly what you're doing. As you gain experience, you might be able to estimate what a pound looks like, but even the most experienced tend to drift up or down in measuring. It's good to know how much you're really feeding your animal even if you're a casual sort.

Scales are inexpensive and easy to use. Set your scale to "pounds and ounces" instead of "grams and kilograms" or you'll be confused! Measurements may be done in cups but it's easy to be off by a few ounces using cups. That's a lot for a medium to small dog or a cat.

A food processor will puree your vegetables and fruits. Dogs and cats don't have sufficient enzymes to digest the cellulose that is the cell wall of veggies and fruits, so we puree them to make it easier for the digestive process to take place (in the ancestral diet, most veggie and fruit content would be pre-digested). When the puree is frozen, this cell wall is further broken down by the action of water expanding as it freezes.

Organ meats are quickly chopped and pureed in the food processor for easier handling, whether you are mixing into a larger quantity of meat or freezing small portions for use in daily meals.

High-powered blenders like the Vita-Mix® or a regular blender work very well for veggies, but a food processor can do the liver chopping with no fuss.

A freezer soon becomes more than a luxury for those who make their own food, unless you like "cooking" every day. Space in our houses is often in short supply, but even a very small freezer can help you be efficient and thrifty. If you want to take advantage of the savings to be gained by buying in bulk, you need a freezer. We all know dog people who consider a crate to be a great end table — you may find that a small freezer is a good counter surface for your kitchen. However you manage it, a freezer will make your life easier.

Buy a freezer thermometer and check the temperature of your freezer regularly. It should be able to maintain 0°. If it doesn't, it isn't working properly. Frost-free freezers cycle through several stages in maintaining themselves and are not as energy efficient as those with manual defrost, but both frost-free and manual defrost freezers should maintain this temperature. Refrigerator freezers don't consistently do this. Though some refrigerator freezers can get to 0°, the intricacies of providing both frozen and refrigerated storage sometimes prevent adequate freezer temperatures. If your ice cream stays as hard as a rock in your refrigerator freezer, and you never find it soft when you creep into the kitchen in the middle of the night, you're probably good. Have a thermometer inside to be sure. This fluctuation in temperature can really affect the quality of food.

A grinder is helpful for even smaller scale food production. You can throw all your meat ingredients together and grind them in no time. Food processors don't work at all for this job. If you use boneless meats, a $100 grinder will suffice, but it may not last long. Some people swear by them, but they're slow and not very powerful. You can feed your meats and organs cut up and mixed with veggies, but the veggies are more palatable mixed with ground meat. There are ways to get around the grinder issue, but a grinder makes food preparation much faster.

If you want to grind turkey necks, or take advantage of great bargains like whole turkeys or chickens, you will need a heavy-duty grinder. This is a major purchase. It's heavy. You need a place to keep it. But there's no denying that if you're making large quantities of food, a grinder really speeds things up. Our current grinder has fed three to five households of critters for over six years and is worn but in great shape.

Check Cabela's® catalog for a starting place. The grinder option with the bigger neck (1 ½ HP) gives you more flexibility for larger bony parts. With the next model down (1 HP), the power is sufficient but you can't get turkey backs in easily.

If you are sure you will never want to grind up a turkey or chicken, and you're only using boneless meats, then a smaller grinder will do. But the $100.00 version will be slow, and if you have big dogs it probably won't last very long.

A quick search on the internet will find you many opinions and options.

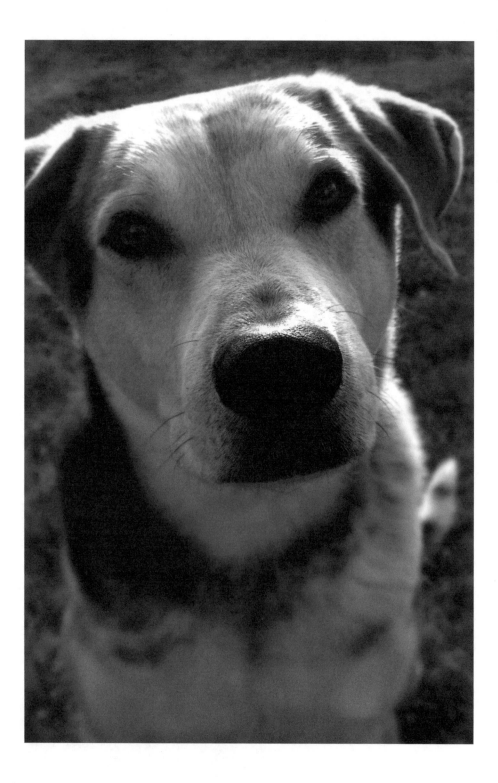

RECIPES, FEEDING CHARTS AND TRANSITION

The first recipe section in this chapter covers veggie and fruit mixes. They are used for both cats and dogs in differing proportions.

The second section is divided into cat and dog segments. Recipe proportions are slightly different. General considerations for cats and dogs are not quite the same either – some have to do with physiology and some have to do with temperament and personality.

The large meat mix recipes make about 10 pounds. This is a manageable amount to prepare and store. This amount provides food for a medium size dog for about seven to ten days, assuming that the dog eats about 1.25 pounds (meat mix with veggies) per day. If you have smaller dogs, it might last ten days (small dogs burn more food for their size, generally). However, meat will not last that long in the refrigerator. Food that can't be used in a few days must be frozen. If you'd rather do the whole thing on a daily basis, or you have very small animals, the smaller recipes may suit you better. A small recipe provides one day's food for most medium size dogs or about 4 meals for a cat.

Organ meats are great sources of minerals and vitamins. They are mixed in with the muscle meat. The fragrance and texture of liver isn't very popular with most humans, so we think it's easier and more pleasant to mix liver and heart into a large amount of meat than to deal with a daily preparation event. You could also prepare organs in portion sizes and add them as you go.

Some organ meats are hard to find, though as you get more experienced you will find sources. If you can't find chicken heart or turkey heart and liver, you can buy freeze-dried organs online from *Fresh is Best Pet Food* or *Bravo* (there may be others). These companies give you the fresh and freeze dried weight equivalents. Some companies also sell organs frozen. You might have to buy direct or order from your pet food retailer, since these products may not be stocked even if the brand is carried.

In this new edition, we're more flexible about this issue. We have modified some of the recipes to include revised amounts of organs that are easy to find. If you're persistent and can get all the matching organs for the original recipes, we're very happy about that. But the revised recipes work well, too.

Meat may be cut up or ground. Organ meats may also be cut up rather than ground. If you are chopping, it's easier to mix everything evenly if you chop the organs into pieces and chop them smaller in the food processor. Some pets do better with their organ meats ground than with whole pieces. For example, one of our dogs regurgitates large pieces of heart but has no problem when they're ground.

Feeding meat in chunks is good for both dental hygiene and exercise for cats and for dogs who are inclined to chew rather than gulp. Chewing and shearing meat is a very satisfying experience for carnivores! However, if your enthusiastic carnivore swallows chunks whole, there will be no benefit, and sometimes chunks will be regurgitated.

Recipes with bone meal or other calcium/phosphorus powder may be cooked lightly if that is your preference. A meal or a batch can be gently baked or simmered just until the meat changes color. That's enough!

DO NOT COOK RECIPES WITH RAW GROUND BONE.

Unless ground bone is very, very finely ground, so fine that it is almost invisible to the eye and the fingers feel only smoothness, it can become sharp and brittle when cooked.

The veggie and fruit ingredients may be varied, as discussed earlier, but don't increase the starchy vegetables much, because you will add carbohydrate and change the nutrition profile. If you increase the other veggies much, you'll reduce the calorie count – and change the nutrition profile. Though there are some good medical reasons to feed a higher veggie diet this should be done with medical supervision.

Veggie mix recipes are sized so that they can be mixed with one full meat mix recipe. For dogs, mix a full large meat mix recipe with a large veggie mix recipe. For cats, mix a full small meat mix recipe with a small veggie mix recipe. This is a convenient way to make larger quantities of pre-mixed food, but assumes that you are making both meat mix and veggies on the same day. When you get some experience, you'll have an opinion on this topic. The small recipes are in the same proportions.

The average calorie count of our recipe for cats is 40 calories per ounce and for dogs 35 calories per ounce. For bigger animals, small changes in volume don't make a huge difference. You can adjust as you go with our feeding chart. For small dogs and cats it can be very important to know how many calories you're feeding. For example, an eight-pound mature cat needs about 240 calories a day, so it's easy to figure out that this cat needs about 6 – 7 ounces of food. An ounce is only about 2 tablespoons of food. With a small animal, a little more or a little less makes a difference!

If you trade off with commercial foods, be aware that commercial foods may have higher or lower calorie counts than our program – check each product.

You may have to increase or decrease amounts accordingly!

You can mix your meat, organs and veggies together, or you can prepare them separately and mix together at the time of feeding. The options we offer are just starting places and you'll find ways that work for you. Meat keeps better long-term (more than a couple of months frozen) than produce. If you are making a very large quantity of food, it's probably best to store the meat mix and veggie puree separately. The enzymes in the veggies and fruit will continue to act — slowly — because the food is raw. Veggie puree stored more than a month or two will lose flavor and quality due to this action.

Fatty acid supplements and other perishable additions are best added at meal times. Additions like psyllium or pumpkin might be added for a specific purpose but not on a daily basis, so they should also be added at the time of feeding, as needed.

You may be told that balance over time is good and you don't have to feed everything every day. Our experience is that we humans aren't very good at keeping track of "balance over time." In terms of practical application and accuracy, it's simpler to include everything at every meal when it's possible.

EVERY MEAL =

Meat mix (sometimes with eggs, sardines or salmon)
+ Veggie/fruit mix
+ Bone meal or bone
+ Mineral and vitamin supplement
+ Fatty acid supplement (may not be every meal)

SOME TERMS AND ABBREVIATIONS

To accurately measure cups, ingredients must be chopped, pureed or ground first and then mixed. Or, you can weigh everything on a food scale and mix and puree it all afterward. Whatever works for you is fine. Small amounts and additions given as "teaspoons" (t) or "tablespoons" (T) are small enough quantities to be accurate and need not be weighed.

For cups, use dry measure cups. When they are filled and leveled, the volume that fits in the cup will be very close to the weight desired.

"Scant" means "a little less than." It's hard to be precise when using cups for small quantities, but that "little less than" adds up for small animals. Where space is limited, this is written as "-"(minus).

In the same category is "plus." "1 c +" means a level measuring cup that's a little rounded. Again, this may be only a tablespoon more, but it might be important for a small animal. To save space, we often refer to "plus" as "+."

t = level measuring teaspoon	# = pound (16 oz)
T = level measuring tablespoon	oz = ounce
c = level measuring cup	g = gram
	mg = milligram

1# = 16 oz (ounces) = 2 c
½# = 8 oz (ounces) = 1 c

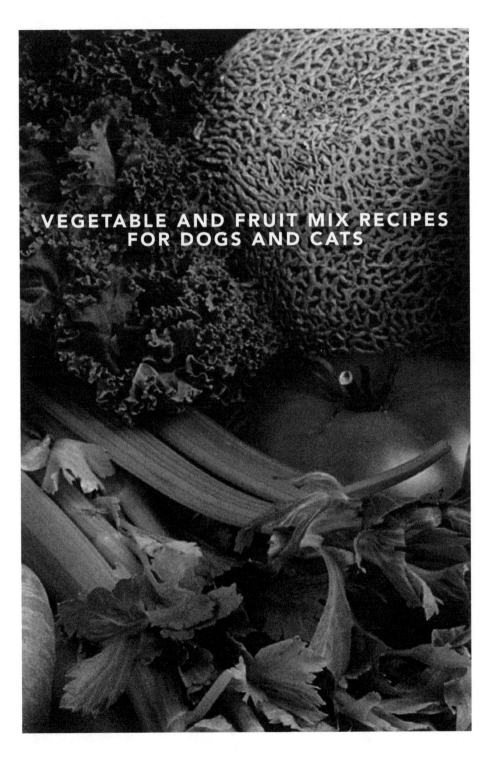

VEGETABLE AND FRUIT MIX RECIPES
FOR DOGS AND CATS

The following recipes are suggestions only. They're combinations that go well together and ones that have the relatively low carbohydrate balance we're suggesting for our basic program. These are the mixes used when we analyzed our program, but there's an infinite variety that will work.

These can be made in large or small batches depending on your need. Those with small animals will do best with the small recipes since raw produce has a limited freezer life.

Feel free to substitute pumpkin and other winter squash or sweet potato (well cooked) in any veggie mix to make up the total amount given, as long as you include most of the lower carbohydrate, bright green, yellow and red ingredients in the recipes. Sweet potatoes especially can add needed calories for a dog that uses a lot of food. However, the phytonutrients provided by the other fruits and vegetables are needed, too.

For all recipes, wash the produce and drain. Discard rinds of melons and winter squash. Puree the ingredients in batches that are small enough to allow your blender to work well. You might have to add a little water.

We've given you instructions in the proportion charts for mixing veggies with meat mix at the time you feed your pets and/or for mixing quantities up to 6 cups of food.

If you prefer to mix big batches of food, these recipes provide the amount to mix with an entire meat mix recipe.

For dogs – mix a large recipe with the entire meat mix recipe

For cats – mix a small recipe with the entire meat mix recipe

If you choose to use other veggies and fruits to make your own veggie mix recipe, use the below proportions.

For dogs – use 7 cups veggie mix for each large meat mix recipe

For cats – use 3 ½ cups veggie mix for each large meat mix recipe

Veggie and fruit recipe #1 – for dogs and cats

Goes well with beef

Large recipe – makes about 7 cups

2 #	(4 c) chopped broccoli
12 oz	(1 ½ c) celery
6 oz	(¾ c) blueberries
6 oz	(¾ c) watermelon

Small recipe – makes about 3 ½ cups

1 #	(2 c) broccoli
6 oz	(¾ c) celery
3 oz	(¼ c + 2 T) blueberries
3 oz	(¼ c + 2 T) watermelon

Veggie and fruit recipe #2 – for dogs and cats

Goes well with chicken

Large recipe – makes about 7 cups

1 #	(2 c) carrots
1 #	(2 c) Chinese cabbage (napa)
1 #	(2 c) red or orange peppers
8 oz	(1 c) cantaloupe

Small recipe – makes about 3 ½ cups

8 oz	(1 c) carrots
8 oz	(1 c) Chinese cabbage (napa)
8 oz	(1 c) red or orange peppers
4 oz	(½ c) cantaloupe

Veggie and fruit recipe #3 – for dogs and cats

Good with turkey

Large recipe – makes about 7 cups

1 ½ #	(3 c) zucchini
8 oz	(1 c) apple
1 ½ #	(3 c) cooked sweet potato

Small recipe – makes about 3 ½ cups

12 oz	(1 ½ c) zucchini
4 oz	(½ c) apple (or unsweetened applesauce)
12 oz	(1 ½ c) cooked sweet potato

CATS

Meat mix recipes – add bone meal 60
    Chicken with liver
    Turkey with liver
    Beef with heart and liver
    Chicken with heart and liver
    Turkey with heart and liver

Meat mix recipes – with ground bone included 65
    Chicken with ground bone, heart and liver
    Turkey with ground bone, heart and liver

Putting the pieces together 68
    Rotation example
    Proportions
        Proportions for meat and veggie meals
        Egg additions
            About egg additions
            Proportions for meals with egg additions
        Sardine or salmon additions
            About sardine and salmon additions
            Proportions for meals with sardine/salmon additions
    Essential additions
        Calcium
        Fatty acids
    Feeding chart
    Successful switching for cats

CATS

MEAT MIX RECIPES – ADD BONE MEAL

Boneless chicken with liver for CATS

Large recipe

9 #   (18 c) lean chicken thighs, with some skin but not much

1 #   (2 c) chicken liver

Small recipe

14.5 oz   (1 ¾ c + 1 T) lean chicken thighs, no skin

 1.5 oz   (3 T) chicken liver

Grind or chop meat and liver. Mix meat and organs well. Use about 10% gizzards as part of the 9# of meat if you can.

The small meat mix recipe makes perhaps 2 or 3 days worth of food for a medium size adult cat. Cats are fussy about freshness. You may need to freeze even small recipes in meal-size portions to maintain freshness, and add veggies at the time of feeding.

Freeze in convenient amounts to use within a day or two after thawing.

 Add supplements at mealtimes

   Calcium source (bone replacement)

   Mineral/vitamin supplement

   Fatty acid supplement (may not be daily depending on product)

7 parts meat mix to 1 part veggies = ⅞ c meat mix + ⅛ c veggies

Add enzymes, glandular, probiotics and other supplements at mealtimes as well, using product guidelines. See our "Optimizing" chapter for more information.

Use your cat's personalized diet card to prevent "diet drifting!"

Boneless turkey with liver for CATS

Large recipe

9 #   (18 c) lean turkey thighs, with some skin but not much

1 #   (2 c) chicken liver (turkey liver if you can get it)

Small recipe

14.5 oz   (1 ¾ c + 1 T) lean turkey thighs, with some skin but not much

1.5 oz   (3 T) chicken liver (turkey liver if you can get it)

Grind or chop meat and liver. Mix meat and organs well. Use about 10% gizzards as part of the 9# of meat if you can.

The small meat mix recipe makes perhaps 2 or 3 days worth of food for a medium size adult cat. Cats are fussy about freshness. You may need to freeze even small recipes in meal-size portions to maintain freshness, and add veggies at the time of feeding.

Freeze in convenient amounts to use within a day or two after thawing.

Add supplements at mealtimes

Calcium source (bone replacement)

Mineral/vitamin supplement

Fatty acid supplement (may not be daily depending on product)

7 parts meat mix to 1 part veggies = ⅞ c meat mix + ⅛ c veggies

Add enzymes, glandular, probiotics and other supplements at mealtimes as well, using product guidelines. See our "Optimizing" chapter for more information.

Use your cat's personalized diet card to prevent "diet drifting!"

Boneless beef with heart and liver for CATS

Large recipe

8.75 #	(17 ½ c) beef, 90-93% lean
1 #	(2 c) beef heart
.25 #	(½ c) beef liver

Small recipe

14 oz	(1 ¾) c beef, 90-93% lean
1.5 oz	(3 T) beef heart
.5 oz	(1 T) beef liver

Grind or chop meat and organs. Mix meat and organs well.

The small meat mix recipe makes perhaps 2 or 3 days worth of food for a medium size adult cat. Cats are fussy about freshness. You may need to freeze even small recipes in meal-size portions to maintain freshness, and add veggies at the time of feeding.

Add supplements at mealtimes

Calcium source (bone replacement)

Mineral/vitamin supplement

Fatty acid supplement (may not be daily depending on product)

7 parts meat mix to 1 part veggies = ⅞ c meat mix + ⅛ c veggies

Add enzymes, glandular, probiotics and other supplements at mealtimes as well, using product guidelines. See our "Optimizing" chapter for more information.

Use your cat's personalized diet card to prevent "diet drifting!"

Boneless chicken with heart and liver for CATS

Large recipe

7.5 #	(15 c) lean boneless chicken thighs with some skin
1 #	(2 c) chicken heart
.5 #	(1 c) chicken liver
1 #	(2 c) chicken gizzards (if you don't use gizzards use 1# more meat)

Small recipe

13 oz	(1½ c + 2T) lean chicken thighs or breasts with some skin (use about 10% gizzards if available)
2 oz	(¼ c) chicken heart
1 oz	(2 T) chicken liver

Boneless chicken thighs and breasts can save you a lot of work. If your pieces still have the bone in, weigh or measure after deboning. Grind or chop meat and organs. Mix well.

The small recipe makes perhaps 2 or 3 days worth of food for a medium size adult cat. Cats are fussy about freshness. You may need to freeze even small recipes in meal-size portions to maintain freshness, and add veggies at the time of feeding.

Add supplements at mealtimes
Calcium source (bone replacement)
Mineral/vitamin supplement
Fatty acid supplement (may not be daily depending on product)

7 parts meat mix to 1 part veggies = ⅞ c meat mix + ⅛ c veggies

Add enzymes, glandular, probiotics and other supplements at mealtimes as well, using product guidelines. See our "Optimizing" chapter for more information.

Use your cat's personalized diet card to prevent "diet drifting!"

Boneless turkey with heart and liver for CATS

Large recipe

7.5 #	(15 c) boneless turkey thigh and breast meat
1 #	(2 c) turkey heart
1 #	(2 c) turkey gizzards (if you don't use gizzards use 1# more meat)
.5 #	(1 c) turkey liver

Small recipe

13 oz	(1 ½ c) lean turkey thigh or breast (use about 10% gizzards if available)
2 oz	(¼ c) turkey heart
1 oz	(2 T) turkey liver

Turkey breasts can be great bargains, but don't use just breast meat – your mix will have less minerals and fat than the plan. At least half thigh meat is good. If your pieces have bone, weigh or measure after deboning. Grind or chop meat and organs. Mix meat and organs well.

The small recipe makes perhaps 2 or 3 days worth of food for a medium size adult cat. Cats are fussy about freshness. You may need to freeze even small recipes in meal-size portions to maintain freshness, and add veggies at the time of feeding.

Add supplements at mealtimes
  Calcium source (bone replacement)
  Mineral/vitamin supplement
  Fatty acid supplement (may not be daily depending on product)

7 parts meat mix to 1 part veggies = ⅞ c meat mix + ⅛ c veggies

Add enzymes, glandular, probiotics and other supplements at mealtimes as well, using product guidelines. See our "Optimizing" chapter for more information.

Use your cat's personalized diet card to prevent "diet drifting!"

RECIPES WITH GROUND BONE FOR CATS

The poultry recipes that follow are a "next step" for those who wish to include fresh bone in their cat food. The proportions give you the proper ratio of bone to meat.

Do not cook recipes with whole or ground bone.

If you make chicken food with bone, a 1 HP (horsepower) grinder will do. If you make turkey food with bone, you need a larger grinder to handle the larger bones. You don't see a beef recipe with bone because beef bones are too hard to grind in a home grinder of any sort. Beef bones are not an appropriate size for cats.

A bone (calcium/phosphorus) supplement is not included in these recipes. Necks provide calcium and phosphorus needed. Because a cat's dietary bone requirement is different than that of a dog, the proportions in the cat recipes are different from those in the dog recipes. As with the boneless recipes, veggie purees can be added to your meat mix when you make it, or added in appropriate amounts when you feed your cat. These recipes were calculated for all life stages.

We prefer for this simple program that you just grind your food with bone, but you may choose to use our proportions to feed whole chicken necks to your animals (do not feed whole turkey necks to cats). If you choose to keep necks whole, make sure that you include the proper amount of meat and organs specified in the rest of the recipe. Refer to the "meat with bone" discussion in the appendix about adding raw bone to your animal's diet, and to our DVD, *Fast Fresh Functional Food for Furry Friends* for an in-depth discussion.

Don't feed whole meals of chicken necks or other bony parts!

Whole birds also give you a good balance of bone to meat. Disjointing chickens for grinding is a large, messy project. Turkeys, being bigger, require the use of more muscle power and a large cleaver to get pieces small enough to fit in the (large) grinder. Give them a try if you have the equipment and you're inclined. You can make food very cheaply this way. If you grind whole birds, add together the weight of the meat and neck amounts in each recipe and use that amount of ground-up bird for the meat portion of the meat mix recipe — you still add the same amount of organs.

There are no small recipes for with bone meat mixes.

Chicken with bone, heart and liver for CATS
DO NOT COOK THIS MIX!

Large recipe
- **4.5 #**   (9 c ground) chicken necks, skinless
- **4 #**   (8 c ground) boneless chicken thigh
- **1 #**   (2 c ground) chicken heart
- **.5 #**   (1 c ground) chicken liver

Grind necks, and chop or grind other ingredients. Mix well. Replace 1# of the boneless meat in the recipe with gizzards if you can.

Add supplements at mealtimes
NO calcium supplement for with bone recipes
Mineral/vitamin supplement
Fatty acid supplement (may not be daily depending on product)

7 parts meat mix to 1 part veggies = ⅞ c meat mix + ⅛ c veggies

Add enzymes, glandular, probiotics and other supplements at mealtimes as well, using product guidelines. See our "Optimizing" chapter for more information.

Use your cat's personalized diet card to prevent "diet drifting!"

Note: yes, the proportions of necks and muscle meat are different in chicken and turkey recipes.

Turkey with bone, liver and heart for CATS
DO NOT COOK THIS MIX!

Large recipe

4 #   (8 c ground) turkey necks, skinless – always grind for cats!

4.5 #   (9 c ground) turkey breast, boneless thigh

1 #   (2 c ground) turkey heart

.5 #   (1 c ground) turkey liver

Grind necks, and chop or grind other ingredients. Mix well. Replace 1# of the boneless meat in the recipe with gizzards if you can.

Add supplements at mealtimes
NO calcium supplement for recipes with bone recipes
Mineral/vitamin supplement
Fatty acid supplement (may not be daily depending on product)

7 parts meat mix to 1 part veggies = ⅞ c meat mix + ⅛ c veggies

Add enzymes, glandular, probiotics and other supplements at mealtimes as well, using product guidelines. See our "Optimizing" chapter for more information.

Use your cat's personalized diet card to prevent "diet drifting!"

Note: yes, the proportions of necks and muscle meat are different in chicken and turkey recipes.

PUTTING THE PIECES TOGETHER

The following pages show you measurements for the components of your cat's diet.

- The meal tables show you the main ingredients.
- The "additions" tables that follow show you the bone meal and fatty acid components.
- Refer to Appendix I for a recipe for a homemade mineral supplement, purchase our product, or find one that meets your cat's needs using the analysis charts. Be aware that most pet products are not sufficient!
- We've planned the rotation assuming two meals a day.

We suggest that you assemble all the pieces on paper (your cat's diet card) so you don't have to refer to the charts on a daily basis.

The meal tables that follow show you proportions to use to make meals for your cat. You can mix up a meal's worth or a few day's worth (if your cat agrees). If it's more convenient for you, you can mix up a couple of month's worth of meat and veggies, but add the eggs and sardines or salmon to meals when you feed your cat.

There is a set of tables for each version of main ingredients:

    meat and veggies

    meat and veggies plus eggs

    meat and veggies plus sardines or salmon

These proportions can be noted on your cat's diet card and you won't need to refer to the tables again.

We've given measurements for those who like to use cups and measuring spoons, and measurements for those who prefer to use a scale. If you're a measuring spoon sort and you've never used a scale, it's worth trying. Measuring spoons can vary widely. Measuring cups (dry measure) are more accurate. A scale is easy to use, easy to clean, and accurate.

Containers vary widely too. When we make large quantities of food, we might use 50 containers of (supposedly) exactly the same size, but when we weigh them there's quite a bit of variation, sometimes up to ½ pound for a 2 pound container. So, there's some true benefit to actually weighing your food. Even if you don't choose to do that, and you come up with a shortcut, check your weights now and then to make sure you're getting close.

After a few days or weeks, you'll develop a good sense of what the specific amount looks like, and you will probably be able to dispense with measuring except now and then, to check that you haven't drifted away from the amount you're supposed to be making. This sounds a bit unlikely, but it's very possible. We have one Labrador who puts on or loses weight pretty easily so occasionally we say "oh, give her a little less" (or more) and shortly we're saying "isn't she a little skinny??" We have lots of experience with this, which is why we recommend that after you get your "eyeballing" skills down, you still check now and then.

There are lots of places where "2 T" is added or removed – that's an ounce. After you've been doing this a while, you'll find a way to "eyeball" this fairly accurately. We find, for example, that you can pile an ounce onto a half cup measuring cup and have it be rounded. So if you weigh that amount and it is indeed the weight you want, you're freed from having to weigh your meat mix every time you feed your cat. Or you might find the ideal container on your shelf.

When you add eggs and sardines or salmon to meals your meat mix is reduced by 25% to allow for the 25% eggs or sardines. The proportion charts follow the ones for just meat and veggie meals.

ROTATION

Below is a sample of a meal rotation with eggs and sardines or salmon added to meat meals. The proportion of meat meals should be 4-5 chicken meals, 4-5 turkey meals, and 5 beef meals (this balance assumes that you feed twice a day, which makes 14 meals a week).

Our rotation includes eggs and sardines with some meat meals. Our rotation spreads out ¼ the total amount of eggs and sardines into 4 meals each. We've varied the meals to which eggs and sardines are added, so that some meat meals have eggs or sardines added with some meals left as just meat and veggie mix.

We think it makes better sense to spread these ingredients through the week. Though the nutrients from fat we get in these foods can be stored by the body, it's probably better to ingest them more than once a week.

In case you're wondering why we put the eggs in the morning and the sardines at night — it's only that many of us humans are also eating eggs in the morning.

	Day 1	Day 2	Day 3	Day 4	Day 5	Day 6	Day 7
AM	Beef	Chicken	Beef + Egg	Turkey + Egg	Chicken	Chicken + Egg	Beef + Egg
PM	Turkey+ Sardines or Salmon	Beef	Chicken + Sardines or Salmon	Chicken	Beef + Sardines or Salmon	Turkey	Turkey + Sardines or Salmon

In the real world it is often more convenient to feed one protein source several days in a row. This is fine. Make sure to get the eggs and sardines into the rotation.

Some people find it easier to measure by weight, some by volume. We've given you both.

MEAT MIX AND VEGGIE MEALS

Proportions for meat and veggie meals for cats

BY VOLUME (cups + tablespoons)

CAT	Meat mix + Veggies (meals with no eggs or sardines)	
To make	Meat mix needed	Veggie mix needed
½ c food	½ c minus 1 T	1 T
1 c food	¾ c + 2 T	2 T
1 ½ c food	1 ¼ c plus 1 T	3 T
2 c food	1 ¾ cup	¼ c

BY WEIGHT (ounces + pounds)

CAT	Meat mix + Veggies (meals with no eggs or sardines)	
To make	Meat mix needed	Veggie mix needed
½ c food	3.5 oz	.5 oz
1 c food	7 oz	1 oz
1 ½ c food	10.5 oz	1.5 oz
2 c food	14 oz	2 oz

EGG ADDITIONS TO CAT MEALS

About egg additions to meals

Eggs are an important contribution to the fatty acid profile of this program. They provide great protein at unbeatable prices.

Eggs may be fed lightly cooked or raw. If you are concerned that raw egg whites may interfere with biotin absorption, cook the eggs slightly so that whites are cooked. Eggs are best cooked over easy, or soft cooked. When the yolk stays uncooked and unbroken, all the fragile fatty acids are preserved.

If you are concerned about bacteria, you may cook eggs to kill possible bacteria. In this case, cook the yolk until it is solid. Eggs are best eaten as soon as they are cooked.

Substantial numbers of animals we know don't digest raw eggs well, but do fine with them cooked. There are lots of possible reasons for this – but we think that if you cook eggs for those who throw up raw eggs or won't eat them raw, eggs will probably still be a good inclusion for your program. This is something you'll learn as you go.

In this edition, we show you how to add eggs to meals over a week rather than giving entire meals of eggs. The sample rotation shows you how many meals should include eggs. Use the tables that follow for proportions of meat mix, veggies and eggs.

Including eggs in cat meals

It's hard to be precise with eggs! There are USDA standards – but real eggs often differ from the standard, and there's a range of weight that's acceptable.

To test our recipes, we bought 6 different brands of large eggs. We weighed them (with and without shells) and measured the results in measuring cups. There was significant difference, up to a half ounce per egg. When weighing 5 eggs, that difference added up to (plus or minus) almost two ounces. We've rounded up or down a bit on the chart that just lists a number of eggs, getting as close as we could.

We've given you ounces in a separate chart to use if you prefer to figure it out that way. Once you get this measurement established, you won't have to think about it again. Also remember, a little more or less isn't going to be a problem unless it's always a little less or always a little more.

Proportions for including eggs in cat meals

BY VOLUME (cups + tablespoons)

CAT	Meat mix + Eggs + Veggies		
To make	Meat mix needed	Eggs needed	Veggie mix needed
½ c food	¼ c + 1 rounded T	½ egg	1 T
1 c food	½ c + 2 rounded T	1 egg	2 T
1 ½ c food	1 c	1 – 2 eggs	3 T
2 c food	1 ¼ c + 1 T	2 eggs	¼ c

BY WEIGHT (ounces + pounds)

CAT	Meat mix + Eggs + Veggies		
To make	Meat mix needed	Eggs needed	Veggie mix needed
½ c food	2.6 oz	.9 oz	.5 oz
1 c food	5.25 oz	1.75 oz	1 oz
1½ c food	7.9 oz	2.6 oz	1.5 oz
2 c food	10.5 oz	3.5 oz	2 oz

Cooked eggs are accepted and tolerated better than raw by the cats we know. Start adding very slowly for best results.

Given the variations we found between eggs when working on these proportions, it might be worth measuring or weighing some eggs to see how yours compare. If they are a lot smaller or bigger it could affect the outcome.

SARDINE AND SALMON ADDITIONS TO CAT MEALS

About sardine and salmon additions to meals

Sardines and wild-caught salmon are an integral part of our program. They provide essential fatty acids and they provide most of the vitamin D that's needed. Without them, your pet's diet would be deficient in vitamin D. Sardines and salmon are a relatively low-cost, real food way to provide this essential nutrient. Currently (2013), it seems likely that genetically modified salmon will be approved by the FDA. We recommend making sure that all your ingredients are GMO free.

If you've never fed your cat sardines or salmon, start slowly. This is fat-rich, calorie-dense food. Start by offering a small piece of sardine or salmon. If all goes well, with no digestive upsets, increase the amounts. For animals who have any history of a problem with fat, starting slowly is prudent.

Cats with addictive personalities could decide to eat only sardines. Though they may love a whole meal of sardines, in the long run it's not a good plan.

Sardines and canned salmon are very convenient. Open the can and serve! Be aware that cats may have opinions about foods that have been opened and refrigerated. Storage of leftovers in glass jars with plastic lids has been our best tactic with this problem.

You may substitute frozen raw sardines or frozen ground sardines (made by raw pet food companies). Buy canned sardines in water. Sardines packed in oil can be drained, but the oils used are not the best quality and many calories are added to a meal even if the oil is drained. The recipes are computed on drained weight, but you can include the water.

For salmon, we recommend that you use canned products. If you use fresh salmon, always cook it because of the possible parasites it might carry. The bones in fresh cooked salmon must be removed because they're brittle. We have included the bone in canned fish products in analyzing the diets. Occasional meals including fresh cooked boneless salmon filets wouldn't upset this balance very much, but if this were always the case the bone meal level would need to be adjusted.

CATS

In our meal charts we include the equivalent of one meal of sardines or salmon per week spread over the week by including it with various meat meals (this amount assumes that you feed your animals twice a day).

Proportions for including sardines or salmon in cat meals

BY VOLUME (cups + tablespoons)

CAT	Meat mix + Sardines or Salmon + Veggies		
To make	Meat mix needed	Sardines needed	Veggie mix needed
½ c food	¼ c + 1 rounded T	¼ can	1 T
1 c food	½ c + 2 rounded T	½ can	2 T
1 ½ c food	1 c	¾ can	3 T
2 c food	1 ¼ c + 1 T	1 can	¼ c

BY WEIGHT (ounces + pounds)

CAT	Meat mix + Sardines or Salmon + Veggies		
To make	Meat mix needed	Sardines needed	Veggie mix needed
½ c	2.6 oz	.9 oz	.5 oz
1 c	5.25 oz	1.75 oz	1 oz
1 ½ c	7.9 oz	2.6 oz	1.5 oz
2 c	10.5 oz	3.5 oz	2 oz

Including sardine or salmon in cat meals

Sardines are pretty easy to use. The choices that have only water are limited. Smaller sardines are handy for small animals, but they are often packed in oil. These extra calories aren't needed, and the oils used aren't the oils we want to add. Cats don't mind if they get a piece instead of a whole fish.

For these recipes, we bought examples of the ones that are water packed. Where we live, these included King Oscar, Crown Prince, Brunswick and Chicken of the Sea. Drained weight ranged from 3 to 3.75 ounces. This difference, as with eggs, can add up.

You can also weigh the drained sardines you buy and figure out your proportions using the table that lists proportions by weight.

For salmon, products range from a few ounces to a pound. Divide them up according to the "by weight" table to determine the serving size.

Once you have these serving sizes determined, you can note them on your diet card and never think about it unless you include a new product in your repertoire.

Comparison shopping is advised. At different stores, for the same sardine product, we paid .65 per can or $2.85.

Cats may have strong food preferences! You may need to add sardines or salmon very slowly, so the above guidelines may need to be adjusted – if you need to start with 1/8 teaspoon of any new food (yes, some cats are like this), you'd adjust the meat mix accordingly.

ESSENTIAL ADDITIONS

Calcium additions for cats and kittens

The calcium supplement amount in the following tables is not the entire requirement listed by AAFCO for cats and kittens. It's the requirement minus the amount that's already found in the food. These amounts added to food provide the AAFCO minimum for adult cats or kittens.

Bone meal products range between 20% and 33% calcium. Most bone meal products are acceptable but the serving sizes are different because the percentage of calcium and other minerals differs. It works best for our recipes to narrow that range a little and we've chosen to use products between 24% and 30%. What you see in the serving size columns of each table is what we found in our kitchens with a gram scale and a selection of sensibly shaped measuring spoons. In our kitchens, a level teaspoon weighs about 3 grams. We translated the package directions into grams and then teaspoons for you. We hope one of these choices translates well for you. If you prefer, you can calculate from the table on the opposite page where serving sizes are listed in milligrams. If this is your choice, be sure to calculate the calcium amount, not the total bone meal amount.

We've rounded the fractions of teaspoons up or down a bit. For example, since 2.3 grams would be difficult to measure, we're getting as close as we can. There's some room for a bit more of most minerals and total precision isn't possible when preparing home food. A little more bone meal will be fine.

As you can see on the chart that follows, what this may come down to is whether your measuring spoon is rounded or level, - (minus) and + (plus). If you have really big animals or lots of them, or you mix up lots of food at a time, it's worth figuring out how much you'd put into 5 or 10 pounds and see how that fits into a ¼ cup measuring cup. Sometimes we do this calculation and add bone meal to a large batch of meat mix.

KITTEN BONE MEAL SERVING SIZE

Brand	NOW 30%	KAL 27%	Naturvet 24%
½ c food	½ t -	½ t -	½ t
1 c food	¾ t	¾ t +	1 t
1 ½ c food	1 t	1 t +	1½ t
2 c food	1½ t	1½ t +	2 t

* Do not use calcium supplements with no phosphorus for kittens or with diets that use high fat ingredients (NOT our program – we use lean meats).

CAT BONE MEAL SERVING SIZE

Brand	NOW 30%	KAL 27%	Naturvet 24%
½ c food	¼ t	¼ t	¼ t +
1 c food	½ t -	½ t	½ t +
1 ½ c food	½ t +	½ t +	¾ t +
2 c food	¾ t +	1 t	1 t +

* Do not use calcium supplements with no phosphorus for kittens or with diets that use high fat ingredients (NOT our program – we use lean meats).

Consult your veterinarian about when your kitten is mature enough to switch to the adult standard.

CALCIUM NEEDS FOR KITTENS FOR THIS RECIPE ROTATION ONLY

½ cup food	335 mg
1 cup food	670 mg
1 ½ cup food	1005 mg
2 cups food	1340 mg

CALCIUM NEEDS FOR CATS FOR THIS RECIPE ROTATION ONLY

½ cup food	188 mg
1 cup food	375 mg
1 ½ cup food	563 mg
2 cups food	750 mg

FATTY ACID ADDITIONS FOR CATS

We know that the balance and amount of omega-3 fatty acids is a very important factor in the diets of our animals and ourselves. The level of omega-3 fatty acids needed for any living creature is a controversial topic. Omega-3 fatty acids are very important, but it doesn't take a lot to balance the fatty acids in the diet. There were not huge amounts of DHA and EPA in the ancestral diet.

Common recommendations range up to 1–2 teaspoons per 20 pounds of an animal's body weight, and higher for some medical conditions (like cancer). These recommendations for animals often exceed the NRC's safe upper limit, and are frequently many times greater than those recommended for humans. Product serving sizes often recommend the same amount of a fish oil supplement for a 45# dog (1000 kcal per day), or for a cat, as for a human (2000 kcal per day), and this recommendation is on the low end of what we frequently see. For cats, the quantity needed is so small that a liquid product would certainly be rancid by the time you use it up. If you are using a liquid product for yourself, then it would be appropriate to use it also for your cat.

There are reasons not to overdo fatty acid supplements. In people, consuming more than 3 g of fish oil per day can result in increased bleeding, according to an article published in the American Heart Association's "Circulation." Fish oil appears to decrease platelet aggregation, which leads to decreased clotting and prolonged bleeding time. Very large intakes have been associated with hemorrhagic stroke, nosebleeds and blood in urine. Symptoms of omega-3 overdose can include GI symptoms, including reflux, nausea (increased licking and swallowing), vomiting, belching, cramping and diarrhea. Probably the most notable symptom of too many omega-3's in animal diets pertains to symptoms of unregulated inflammation. Omega-3's, in proper amounts, control inflammation. If overdone, they enhance the inflammation cascade, resulting in symptoms of inflammation (all of the 'itis' conditions) throughout the body.

There's little basis in science for mega-dosing omega-3 fatty acids. For humans, it seems that more than 500 mg. of a fatty acid product is not effectively used. We don't have that information yet for dogs and cats, but we're all mammals and it's likely that we are similar. From a purely practical point of view, these are really expensive products and there's no reason to give more than can be used. From a functional point of view, megadoses can cause harm given to an animal whose metabololic processes aren't the greatest. If the liver can't break these substances down, and the cells can't use them, then functional problems can result.

Cats on real food programs that include salmon or sardines need only small amounts of supplementation for fatty acids. Cats on sub-optimal foods, like dry food, might need more, but amounts still would be less than commonly recommended.

We like krill oil for the phospholipid properties and the astaxanthin content. Krill oils are made by two major manufacturers. Different brands use one or the other. Levels of EPA and DHA differ. The EPA + DHA levels in good fish oils are similar to those of the krill oils with higher levels of these nutrients. These products are not better or worse, just different.

For ease of use, our chart shows you serving sizes based on the combined amount of EPA and DHA and milligrams of krill oil. This information is on all labels. Other ways of computing (total omega-3s, capsule size) are confusing and sometimes information is missing. If one of the choices we give you in the chart works for you, that's the easy choice.

Few fatty acid products have small enough serving sizes to be convenient for daily use. The mercola.com airtight pumpable krill administers 50mg/pump and may be more convenient than puncturing capsules. The table opposite shows how to use capsule products. Liquid fish oils may contain up to 1200 mg of omega-3s and up to 800 mg of combined EPA and DHA per teaspoon. Broken down for most cats, these products result in a serving size of ⅛ teaspoon per WEEK or 1 capsule PER WEEK. You could do this, but we prefer that you spread your fatty acids over more days. You could be less precise and give your cat a drop or two of your capsule and then you take the rest. The Mercola "kid krill" oil product works well for a cat that eats 1 cup of food a day – a very common quantity. For this example, one Mercola "kid" capsule a day is the serving size.

The chart below shows serving sizes based on the amount of food your cat eats per day. If you have multiple cats you can multiply the serving size accordingly, or feed each cat its supplements individually.

FATTY ACIDS: DAILY SERVINGS FOR CATS

Table 1	Daily Serving	Krill Oil	Daily Total
cups food	Mercola kid krill		combined epa + dha
1 c food	1 cap per day	65 – 125 mg	20 mg
2 c food	2 caps per day	125 – 250 mg	40 mg

If you choose a concentrated product, it's best to give it on days when you are not already feeding fish, so that you spread out the fatty acids more. Sample liquid fish oils claim from 800 – 1100 mg combined EPA and DHA in one teaspoon of their product.

FATTY ACIDS: WEEKLY SERVINGS FOR CATS

Table 2	WEEKLY Serving	WEEKLY Serving	WEEKLY Total
cups food	Neptune Krill oil or similar product	Sample fish oil	approximate combined epa + dha desired
1 c food	1 cap per week	⅛ t per week	140 mg
2 c food	2.25 caps per week	¼ t per week	280 mg

HOW MUCH DO I FEED MY CATS?

It seems that there should be an easy way to figure out how much food to feed your cat, but there's not. You need to know your cat and you need to develop some skill in evaluating her condition. There are good charts to help you evaluate whether your cat is thin or fat, but breed type, age and other factors make it more complicated than just looking at a chart.

Different breeds and breed types have different metabolisms. Cat breeds and body types range from the slender and elongated to the stocky and muscular.

Young and old animals of the same size may eat different amounts. Cats mature fairly quickly. Most of their growing is done in the first five months. During this time more food is required per pound. Most kittens do well being fed 3 times daily as much as they desire to eat in 20 minutes. Be aware of the weight and condition of your cat so you can cut back or add food if needed.

Overweight animals should not lose weight too rapidly. Start out feeding them for slightly under their current weight and adjust so that they lose no more than 1 – 2% of their body weight per month. If your cat is obese, enlist assistance from your veterinarian to monitor her health during weight loss and use 1 – 2% of body weight per month as a guide.

Most frequently we see cats that are overweight. For these cats, a change in food that is not well understood might result in too rapid weight loss. This often happens when slightly chubby cats are switched to fresh food. A food switch is often also a big reduction in calorie count, though the volume being fed looks the same. Owners get very enthusiastic about their pet's new waist-line and just keep going. Ribs and spines should not stick out in the healthy, mature cat. Body fat is needed for many important functions.

Old cats with poor muscle tone and decreased muscle mass may be both fat and have bones sticking out, so consult your veterinarian to get an objective opinion.

Cats are often resistant when it comes to diet change. Make sure your cat is transitioning acceptably. Cats must eat daily or they can have terrible meta-bolic problems. Obese cats may do best being weaned off dry food and onto canned food, then off canned food onto homemade cooked food, then onto homemade raw food. Obese cats must be dieted very slowly and with the help and supervision of a veterinarian.

If you are switching your overweight cat from dry food to fresh food, it's common to see a significant weight loss in the first week. This is usually the result of the body letting go of water retained due to the inflammatory effects of grain-based food. It's quite impressive, but future weight loss should take place more gradually.

Your food scale will help you keep track of how much you're really feeding. If you always feed your cat the same amount of food and now he's getting fat or thin, you need to know why, and you need to be sure you know how much you're really giving him.

Is this a seasonal thing? Does he need less food in the summer, more food in the winter, or the reverse? Is he getting food from another source (someone else's bowl) or have you absentmindedly increased the treats? If you're sure you're giving him the same amount, you can look at exercise, activity and other factors in making sure that all is well.

If he's losing weight on the same amount of food, there might be medical trouble brewing — or you might have changed the composition of the food, or conditions have changed, or a product has changed. We know of a cat who lost two pounds in two months when he was switched from a beef food to a turkey food. The beef product had a lot more calories (fat) than the turkey food, and the owner did not allow for this by adjusting the amount of food fed. On the other hand, weight loss occurs in many different health problems, including parasites. Don't ignore unexpected weight loss.

The charts for feeding amounts are given in cups for general guidelines.

The best way to find out what's right for your cat is to start at an appropriate point in the range and see how it goes. Active and young animals start toward the top of the range, and older or chubby animals in the middle. Evaluate you pet's condition frequently! Too much food may cause digestive upset or weight gain. Too little and your cat may become so thin that her body is unable to maintain vital functions.

We recommend that you weigh your cat weekly until you know how much food she needs to maintain weight.

Directions are based on the calorie count of our recipes. We've included the entire range of recommendations in making the charts. Fresh food veterans agree that animals often maintain weight and condition on ⅓ fewer calories than those recommendations.

There really are no fast, easy answers. Only experience will show you what's right for your animal.

The cat recipes average:
40 calories per ounce
640 calories per pound.

This is a little more than the dog recipes. The difference is in the lower veggie content of the cat recipe.

Don't get too attached to the categories on the following page. Your individual cat may stay in the food range of a "moderately active" all his life. Or, he may graduate to the "older/inactive" category when he's two, even though he's pretty active. The amounts are given as a guideline. Each animal is different. "Official" calorie recommendations are based on results with animals eating dry food. In our experience, the results with real food may be quite different.

The volume of food that a young, active cat can eat may seem like a lot. Dry food packs a lot of calories into a cup, and even grain free products include substantial carbohydrate levels. A cup of real food made from lean meats, which has all the water still in it, often has less than half the calories of the cup of dry food. 1 cup of our food has about 300 calories. 1 cup of a regular dry cat food often has more than 500 calories, and sometimes more. You'll get used to the volume of real food, but the actual number of calories your cat consumes may be less than what's recommended — even though it may seem like a lot of food! You need to feed your young growing kitten as much as it takes to maintain condition. Do not increase any one component of the diet for young/growing animals. The diet is balanced for all life stages.

At the other end of the spectrum, our adult, healthy pets maintain their weight eating an amount of food at the low end of the "inactive" category, unless they are very active. If you calculated the calorie count, it wouldn't seem likely that it's enough given the charts, but that's our real life experience. Don't assume it will be your experience, but be aware that it's not unusual.

Suggested range of amounts to feed per day

Divide amount by number of meals fed.
Totals are for meat mixed with veggies.

CAT	Kitten 3 months	Kitten 5 months	Adult Active	Adult Moderately Active	Adult Older/Inactive
2#	1 c				
3#	1 c +	½ c			
4#	1 ½ c	¾ c	¾ c	½ c	⅓ c +
5#			⅞ c	½ c +	½ c scant
7#			1 c +	¾ c	½ c + 1 T
9#			1 ¼ c	1 c scant	¾ c
11#			1 ½ c	1 c + 1 T	⅞ c
13#			1 ¾ c	1 ⅓ c	1 c scant
15#			1 ⅞ c	1 ½ c	1 c

Few 15-17 pound cats are at their proper weight! Help your cat lose extra ounces with veterinary supervision that considers general health and condition, so they lose at a rate that's safe.

SUCCESSFUL SWITCHING FOR CATS

Change your cat over to real food in a way that makes sense to you. It might take a while for you to get comfortable with the whole idea and that's fine – but your animal's body is probably ready for a new concept in food today and you'll be a hero when you start handing out real food. The total switch can often be accomplished within a week. However, we've known cats to take three months or longer to switch.

Eliminate free feeding! The first task for most cat feeders is to stop leaving a bowl of food out. Cats are much more receptive to new foods if they are hungry. Food left out all day gathers unpleasant critters and quickly becomes rancid (smell it if you doubt us). Every time your cat strolls by the food dish the smell of food makes his system think it's about to get food, starting the whole digestive process. This is not a healthy thing. Cats don't need food to prevent them from being a) upset that we left them all day b) a tiny bit hungry c) bored and d) all the other reasons we think of to justify this unhealthy practice. If you continue to free feed your chances of a successful switch to real food are much lower than if you stop free feeding now.

Take up that food bowl! Establish regular feeding times and put the food away between feedings. Start with two meals of dry food (taking the bowl up after each meal) and a snack of real food, and work your way up from there.

Cats frequently have strong opinions about diet changes. It sounds simple to just switch your cat's food — after all, meat tastes better than dry food! Your cat may disagree. Dry foods are designed to be tasty, and many cats are addicted to the salt and fat included. Often, cats are not open to the idea of variety, especially if they have only been fed one food (as we have been advised by pet food companies for decades). Creativity and patience may be needed to switch your cat to a fresh food diet.

Start by feeding your cat a little bit of fresh food and see how she does with it. If all is well, keep increasing, but start taking out some of the old food. If things are going well, you can usually remove the old food within a few days. Another option is to add the new food as a mid-day snack, to see how she handles it. Remember, the main stimulus for cats to try new foods is hunger.

If you need to keep feeding some dry food (for instance if you are gone overnight and you have a feeder with a timer) figure out the appropriate daily amount of fresh food and the daily amount of dry food and use fractions of that daily ration to base your plan on.

For example, Fred eats a half-cup of dry food a day. You calculate that he would eat 8 ounces of fresh food a day. In the morning, feed him 4 ounces (½ cup) of fresh food (half his daily fresh food ration). In the evening, feed him half of his dry food ration (¼ cup) for one meal. It's best to keep the dry food separate from the fresh, uncooked food. This is just one example. Each individual might be treated differently.

Calculate fresh and dry food separately. Dry food and fresh or canned food have very different calorie counts due to the water in wet foods and the absence of water in dry foods. One cup of dry food has many more calories than one cup of fresh or frozen food, which still contains all the natural water. If you're using commercial foods, you must know the calorie count per pound or ounce so that you can be accurate.

Take this difference into consideration, or you might find yourself seriously underfeeding your cat in the process of switching. We have talked to many people who thought that fresh food was bad for their cat because he lost so much weight. In fact, they were still feeding the volume per day that was the cat's dry food ration. When the amount was adjusted and he was fed more, he thrived.

Cats do well with two meals a day. Kittens are fed frequently as babies and less frequently as they mature. Old animals sometimes do better with frequent feedings, as do ill and recovering animals. Otherwise, observe your cat and see what plan you think works best. Try to resist the cat's opinion that he should be fed every 15 minutes.

Cats are not good candidates for the "tough love" approach. They will starve themselves. Some very serious conditions can occur if cats do not eat for an extended period, especially if cats are overweight. A slow switch will prevent problems. Cats must eat daily.

That said, a healthy animal that has an opportunity to become a bit hungry will make the switch more readily. This is one reason that we strongly recommend that you pick up the dry food dish and move immediately to meals at times that are appropriate for your cat. Check with your veterinarian about what's safe for your cat.

Because raw food and canned food have the same consistency, many cats do best weaned onto canned food. Once on canned food, you can slowly mix raw food into canned food (slowly, slowly) and trick them into eating raw food. Slowly for a cat might mean mixing ¼ teaspoon of a new food into a meal. For long-term success, it's better to begin slowly than to have a cat refuse to eat – cats have very long memories.

Offer bits of fresh food that you are eating. Your cats may refuse, but one day… they won't. Your goal is to help your cat to consider eating foods other than dry, crunchy items.

If your pet has loose stools, wait until the stool is firm to continue the transition. If loose stools continue, consult your holistic veterinarian.

There are many medical conditions that are strongly affected by diet. If you want a veterinary opinion that helps you transition your cat to real food, you need to discuss this with a veterinarian who is interested in fresh food diets. Expecting answers that will help you from a dry food supporter is an exercise in frustration.

Many cats come to real food diets because they have GI problems ranging from diarrhea to Inflammatory Bowel Disease or allergies and skin problems. Cats with unhealthy guts may not do well on raw food initially. Don't give up! Cook food to start with, and make a transition to raw food over three months. Food can be a miracle cure — but frequently there are bumps in the road and a holistic practitioner can help a lot.

Feed multiple cats separately. Yes, really. There are reasons to do this related to social dynamics, but the practical reason is that you need to know who is eating what and how much. This is information that's important every day but especially if one of your cats becomes ill or changes her eating habits.

Cat whiskers are very sensitive. If food is served in a bowl that interferes with whiskers, it could be enough to keep the cat from considering the food. A flat dish works well.

Trickery sometimes works with cats. Put the food on YOUR plate, or hide it in a location cats know to be forbidden. Creativity helps!

Cats generally prefer their food between room temperature and body temperature. Warming food releases the flavors and aromas. Cats choose food by smell. Wet food is a lot less fragrant than a dry food they have been eating. This is often the reason that the second half of a can of food that has been refrigerated is refused — the first time it was at room temperature.

The optimum diet for most cats is a well-balanced, meat-based raw or home cooked diet. If your cat is really opposed to raw or home-made food, the next best option is canned food.

If you use canned food, at least your cat's diet will be fully hydrated. You will be much closer to providing him with optimum nutrition than if you feed dry food. Canned foods that approximate the natural diet of a cat are the best choice. They're advertised as "grain-free." Make sure that you buy products that are "complete." In the "grain-free" products you may find products with plenty of sweet potatoes or potatoes or peas, making these foods starchier than we prefer. Check our website for a few current choices that we think have a good protein/fat/carbohydrate balance.

The worst choice for cats (and their kidneys) is dry food, even if the ingredients are impeccable. Cats need food that contains water.

It may sound odd, but it's important to not care too much about the end result both in how you behave and how you think and feel about this. Even though you might know that this is the absolute best thing for your cat, if you make too big a thing of it in your mind or your actions you may set off resistance in your cat. Cats are good at sensing tension. This is sometimes the case with dogs too, but dogs usually say, "Right! Food!" Cats, on the other hand, often say, "You must be joking!"

DOGS

Meat mix recipes – add bone meal 91
  Chicken with liver
  Turkey with liver
  Beef with heart and liver
  Chicken with heart and liver
  Turkey with heart and liver
Meat mix recipes – with ground bone 96
  Chicken with ground bone, heart and liver
  Turkey with ground bone, heart, and liver
Putting the pieces together 100
  Rotation example
  Proportions
    Proportions for meat and veggie meals
    Egg additions
      About egg additions
      Proportions for meals with egg additions
    Sardine or salmon additions
      About sardine and salmon additions
      Proportions for meals with sardine/salmon additions
  Essential additions
    Calcium
    Fatty acids
  Feeding chart
  Successful switching for dogs

MEAT MIX RECIPES – ADD BONE MEAL

Boneless chicken with liver for DOGS

Large recipe

9 #   (18 c) boneless lean chicken thighs, no skin

1 #   (2 c) chicken liver

Small recipe

14.5 oz   (1 ¾ c +) lean boneless chicken thighs, no skin

1.5 oz   (3 T) chicken liver

Grind or chop meat and organs. Mix meat and organs well. Replace 1# of the meat in recipe with gizzards if available.

Freeze in convenient amounts to use within a day or two after thawing.

Add supplements at mealtimes
    Calcium source (bone replacement)
    Mineral/vitamin supplement
    Fatty acid supplement (may not be daily depending on product)

3 parts meat mix to 1 part veggies = 1 ½ c meat mix + ½ c veggies

Add enzymes, glandular, probiotics and other supplements at mealtimes as well, using product guidelines. See our "Optimizing" chapter for more information.

Use your dog's personalized diet card to prevent "diet drifting!"

DOGS

Boneless turkey with liver for DOGS

Large recipe

9 #   (18 c) boneless lean turkey thighs, no skin

1 #   (2 c) chicken liver

Small recipe

14.5 oz   (1 ¾ c +) lean turkey thigh, no skin

1.5 oz   (3 T) chicken liver

Grind or chop meat and organs. Mix meat and organs well. Replace 1# of the meat in the recipe with gizzards if available.

Freeze in convenient amounts to use within a day or two after thawing.

   Add supplements at mealtimes
     Calcium source (bone replacement)
     Mineral/vitamin supplement
     Fatty acid supplement (may not be daily depending on product)

3 parts meat mix to 1 part veggies = 1 ½ c meat mix + ½ c veggies

Add enzymes, glandular, probiotics and other supplements at mealtimes as well, using product guidelines. See our "Optimizing" chapter for more information.

Use your dog's personalized diet card to prevent "diet drifting!"

Boneless beef with liver and heart for DOGS

Large recipe

8 #	(16 c) beef, 90 – 93% lean
1 #	(2 c) beef heart
1 #	(2 c) beef liver

Small recipe

13 oz	(1 ¾ c) beef, 90 – 93% lean
1.5 oz	(3 T) beef heart
1.5 oz	(3 T) beef liver

Grind or chop meat and organs. Mix meat and organs well.

Freeze in convenient amounts to use within a day or two after thawing.

Add supplements at mealtimes
   Calcium source (bone replacement)
   Mineral/vitamin supplement
   Fatty acid supplement (may not be daily depending on product)

3 parts meat mix to 1 part veggies = 1 ½ c meat mix + ½ c veggies

Add enzymes, glandular, probiotics and other supplements at mealtimes as well, using product guidelines. See our "Optimizing" chapter for more information.

Use your dog's personalized diet card to prevent "diet drifting!"

DOGS

Boneless chicken with liver and heart for DOGS

Large recipe

7.5 #	(15 c) lean chicken thighs or breasts with some skin
1 #	(2 c) chicken heart
.5 #	(1 c) chicken liver
1#	(2 c) chicken gizzards (if you don't use gizzards use 1# more meat)

Small recipe

13 oz	(1½ c + 2 T) lean chicken thighs or breasts with some skin (use some gizzards if available)
2 oz	(¼ c) chicken heart
1 oz	(2 T) chicken liver

If your pieces still have the bone in, weigh or measure after deboning. Grind or chop meat and organs. Mix well.

Add supplements at mealtimes
Calcium source (bone replacement)
Mineral/vitamin supplement
Fatty acid supplement (may not be daily depending on product)

3 parts meat mix to 1 part veggies = 1 ½ c meat mix + ½ c veggies

Add enzymes, glandular, probiotics and other supplements at mealtimes as well, using product guidelines. See our "Optimizing" chapter for more information.

Use your dog's personalized diet card to prevent "diet drifting!"

Boneless turkey with liver and heart for DOGS

Large recipe

7.5 #   (15 c) boneless turkey thigh and breast meat

.5 #   (1 c) turkey liver

1 #   (2 c) turkey heart

1 #   (2 c) turkey gizzards (if you don't use gizzards use 1# more meat)

Small recipe

13 oz   (1 ½ c + 2 T) lean turkey thigh or breast
(use some gizzards if available)

2 oz   (¼ c) turkey heart

1 oz   (2 T) turkey liver

If your pieces have bone, weigh or measure after boning. Grind or chop meat and organs. Mix meat and organs well.

Add supplements at mealtimes
Calcium source (bone replacement)
Mineral/vitamin supplement
Fatty acid supplement (may not be daily depending on product)

3 parts meat mix to 1 part veggies = 1 ½ c meat mix + ½ c veggies

Add enzymes, glandular, probiotics and other supplements at mealtimes as well, using product guidelines. See our "Optimizing" chapter for more information.

Use your dog's personalized diet card to prevent "diet drifting!"

DOGS

RECIPES WITH GROUND BONE AND ORGANS FOR DOGS

The poultry recipes that follow are a "next step," for those who wish to include fresh bone in their dog food. The proportions give you the proper ratio of bone to meat.

Do not cook recipes with whole or ground bone.

If you make chicken food with bone, a 1 HP (horsepower) grinder may do. If you make turkey food with bone (or if you move on to whole birds or turkey legs) you need a larger grinder to handle the larger bones. You don't see a beef recipe with bone because beef bones are too hard to grind in a home grinder of any sort. You can feed some whole, raw beef bones but it's hard to estimate proportions, and these bones are loaded with fat and marrow.

We suggest that you stick to the beef recipe with bone meal to ensure that you have the right balance and provide your dog with the occasional recreational knuckle-bone if it's appropriate for your animal – but not often unless you're going to work your dog hard and frequently. A commercial 6-inch marrow bone provides about 1000 calories. Check with your holistic veterinarian about proper bite (tooth alignment) and general health.

A bone (calcium/phosphorus) supplement is not included in these recipes. Necks provide bone. (Because a dog's dietary bone requirement is different than that of a cat, the proportions in these recipes are also different). As with the boneless recipes, veggie purees may be added to your meat mix when you make it, or added in appropriate amounts when you feed your pet. These recipes were calculated for all life stages.

We prefer for this simple program that you grind your food with bone. You may choose to use our proportions to feed whole turkey and chicken necks to your animals. If you choose to keep necks whole, include the proper amount of meat and organs specified in the rest of the recipe. Refer to our DVD, *Fast Fresh Functional Food for Furry Friends* for an in-depth discussion.

Don't feed whole meals of chicken necks or other bony parts!

Whole birds can give you a good balance of bone to meat. Disjointing chickens for grinding is a large, messy project. Turkeys, being bigger, require the use of more muscle power and a large cleaver to get pieces small enough to fit in the (large) grinder. Give them a try if you have the equipment. You can make food very cheaply this way. If you grind whole birds, add together the weight of the meat and neck amounts in each recipe and use that amount of ground-up bird for the meat portion of the meat mix recipe — you still add the organs.

DOGS

Chicken with bone, liver and heart for DOGS
DO NOT COOK THIS MIX!

5.25 #	(10 ½ c ground) chicken necks, skinless
3.25 #	(6 ½ c ground) boneless chicken thigh
.5 #	(1 c ground) chicken heart
.5 #	(1 c ground) chicken liver
.5 #	(1 c ground) chicken gizzard

Grind necks, and chop or grind other ingredients. Mix well.

  Add supplements at mealtimes
    NO calcium addition for recipes with bone
    Mineral/vitamin supplement
    Fatty acid supplement (may not be daily depending on product)

3 parts meat mix to 1 part veggies = 1 ½ c meat mix + ½ c veggies

Add enzymes, glandular, probiotics and other supplements at mealtimes as well, using product guidelines. See our "Optimizing" chapter for more information.

 Use your dog's personalized diet card to prevent "diet drifting!"

Turkey with bone, liver and heart for DOGS
DO NOT COOK THIS MIX!

5.25 #   (10 ½ c ground) turkey necks, skinless

3.25 #   (6 ½ c ground) turkey boneless thigh

  .5 #   (1 c ground) turkey heart

  .5 #   (1 c ground) turkey liver

  .5 #   (1c ground) turkey gizzard

Grind necks, and chop or grind other ingredients. Mix well.

  Add supplements at mealtimes
    NO calcium addition for recipes with bone
    Add mineral/vitamin mix
    Fatty acid supplement (may not be daily depending on product)

3 parts meat mix to 1 part veggies = 1 ½ c meat mix + ½ c veggies

Add enzymes, glandular, probiotics and other supplements at mealtimes as well, using product guidelines. See our "Optimizing" chapter for more information.

Use your dog's personalized diet card to prevent "diet drifting!"

DOGS

PUTTING THE PIECES TOGETHER

The following pages show measurements for the components of your dog's diet.

- The meal tables show you the main ingredients.
- The "additions" tables that follow show you the bone meal and fatty acid components.
- Refer to Appendix I for a homemade mineral supplement, purchase our product, or find one that meets your dog's needs using the analysis charts. Be aware that most pet supplements are not sufficient or appropriate.

We've planned the rotation assuming two meals a day.

We suggest that you assemble all the pieces on paper (your dog's diet card) so you don't have to refer to the charts on a daily basis.

The meal tables that follow show you proportions to use to make meals for your dog. You can mix up a meal's worth or a few day's worth. If it's more convenient for you, you can mix up a couple of month's worth of meat and veggies, but add the eggs and sardines to meals when you feed your dog.

There is a set of tables for each version of main ingredients:
- meat and veggies
- meat and veggies plus eggs
- meat and veggies plus sardines or salmon

These proportions can be noted on your dog's diet card and you won't need to refer to the tables again.

We've given measurements for those who like to use cups and measuring spoons, and measurements for those who prefer to use a scale. If you're a measuring spoon sort and you've never used a scale, it's worth trying. Measuring spoons can vary widely. Measuring cups (dry measure) are more accurate. A scale is easy to use, easy to clean, and accurate.

Containers vary widely too. When we make large quantities of food, we might use 50 containers of (supposedly) exactly the same size, but when we weigh them to be sure there's quite a bit of variation, sometimes up to ½ pound. There's some true benefit to actually weighing your food. Even if you don't choose to weigh your food all the time, and you come up with a shortcut, check your weights now and then to make sure you're getting close.

After a few days or weeks, you'll develop a good sense of what the specific amount looks like, and you will probably be able to dispense with measuring except now and then, to check that you haven't drifted away from the amount you're supposed to be making. This sounds a bit unlikely, but it happens frequently. We have one Labrador who puts on or loses weight pretty easily so occasionally we say "oh, give her a little less" (or more) and shortly we're saying "isn't she a little skinny??." We have lots of experience with this, which is why we recommend that after you get your "eyeballing" skills down, you still check now and then.

There are lots of places where "2 T" is added or removed – that's an ounce. After you've been doing this a while, you'll find a way to estimate fairly accurately. We find, for example, that you can pile an ounce onto a half cup measuring cup and have it be rounded. So if you weigh that amount and it is indeed the weight you want, you're freed from having to weigh your meat mix every time you feed your dog. Or you might find the ideal container on your shelf.

When you're adding eggs and sardines to meals your meat mix is reduced by 25% to allow for the 25% eggs or sardines. The proportion charts follow the chart for just meat and veggie meals.

DOGS

ROTATION

Below is a sample of a meal rotation with eggs and sardines added to meat meals. The meat balance doing meals this way is 4 – 5 chicken 4 – 5 turkey, and 5 beef – we assume that you feed 2 meals a day.

We suggest that you add eggs and sardines to meat meals. This spreads out ¼ the total amount of eggs and sardines into 4 meals each. We've varied the meals to which eggs and sardines are added, so that some of each meat has eggs or sardines added with some meals left as just meat and veggie mix.

We think it makes better sense to spread these ingredients through the week. Though nutrients from fat (the vitamins and fatty acids from these foods) can be stored by the body, it's probably better to ingest them more than once a week.

In case you're wondering why we put the eggs in the morning and the sardines at night – it's only because many of us humans are also eating eggs in the morning.

	Day 1	Day 2	Day 3	Day 4	Day 5	Day 6	Day 7
AM	Beef	Chicken	Beef + Egg	Turkey + Egg	Chicken	Chicken + Egg	Beef + Egg
PM	Turkey+ Sardines or Salmon	Beef	Chicken + Sardines or Salmon	Chicken	Beef + Sardines or Salmon	Turkey	Turkey + Sardines or Salmon

In the real world it is often more convenient to feed one protein source several days in a row. This is fine. Just make sure to get the eggs and sardines into the rotation.

MEAT MIX AND VEGGIE MEALS

Meat mix and veggie proportions for dog meals

BY VOLUME (cups + tablespoons)

DOG	Meat mix + Veggies (meals with no eggs or sardines)	
To make	Meat mix needed	Veggie mix needed
½ c food	⅜ c	⅛ c
1 c food	¾ c	¼ c
2 c food	1 ½ c	½ c
3 c food	2 ¼ c	¾ c
4 c food	3 c	1 c
5 c food	3 ¾ c	1 ¼ c
6 c food	4 ½ c	1 ½ c

BY WEIGHT (ounces + pounds)

DOG	Meat mix + Veggies (meals with no eggs or sardines)	
To make	Meat mix needed	Veggie mix needed
½ c food	3 oz	1 oz
1 c food	6 oz	2 oz
2 c food	12 oz	4 oz
3 c food	1# 2 oz	6 oz
4 c food	1# 8 oz	8 oz
5 c food	1# 14 oz (30 oz)	10 oz
6 c food	2# 4 oz (36 oz)	12 oz

DOGS

EGG ADDITIONS TO DOG MEALS

About egg additions

Eggs are an important contribution to the fatty acid profile of this program. They provide great protein at unbeatable prices.

Eggs may be fed lightly cooked or raw. If you are concerned that raw egg whites may interfere with biotin absorption, cook the eggs slightly so that whites are cooked. Eggs are best cooked over easy, or soft cooked. When the yolk stays uncooked and unbroken, all the fragile fatty acids are preserved. If you are concerned about bacteria, you can cook eggs to kill possible bacteria. In this case, cook the yolk until it is solid. Eggs are best eaten as soon as they are cooked.

Substantial numbers of animals we know don't digest raw eggs well, but do fine with them cooked. There are lots of possible reasons for this. We think that if you cook eggs for those who throw up raw eggs or who refuse to eat them, eggs will probably still be a good inclusion for your program. This is something you'll learn as you go.

In this edition, we show you how to add eggs to meals over a week rather than giving entire meals of eggs. Use the proportion tables that follow to compute your meal proportions, using weight or volume.

Including eggs in dog meals

It's hard to be precise with eggs! There are USDA standards – but real eggs often differ from the standard, and there's a range of weight that's acceptable.

To test our recipes, we bought 6 different brands of large eggs. We weighed them (with and without shells) and measured the results in measuring cups. There was significant difference, up to a half ounce per egg. When weighing 5 eggs, that difference added up to (plus or minus) almost two ounces. We've rounded up or down a bit on the chart that just lists a number of eggs, getting as close as we could.

We've given you ounces in a separate chart to use if you prefer to figure it out that way. Once you get this measurement established, you won't have to think about it again. Also remember, a little more or less isn't going to be a problem unless it's always a little less or always a little more.

Proportions for including eggs in dog meals

BY VOLUME (cups + tablespoons + number of eggs)

DOG	Meat mix + Eggs + Veggies		
To make	Meat mix	Eggs	Veggie mix
½ c food	¼ c + ½ T	½ egg	2 T
1 c food	½ c + 1 T	1 egg	¼ c
2 c food	1 c + 2 T	1 – 2 eggs	½ c
3 c food	1 ½ c + 3 T	2 – 3 eggs	¾ c
4 c food	2 ¼ c	3 – 4 eggs	1 c
5 c food	2 ¾ c + 1 T	4 – 5 eggs	1 ¼ c
6 c food	3⅓ c	5 – 6 eggs	1 ½ c

BY WEIGHT (ounces + pounds)

DOG	Meat mix + Eggs + Veggies		
To make	Meat mix	Eggs	Veggie mix
½ c food	2.25 oz	.75 oz	1 oz
1 c food	4.5 oz	1.5 oz	2 oz
2 c food	9 oz	3 oz	4 oz
3 c food	13.5 oz	4.5 oz	6 oz
4 c food	1# 2 oz (18 oz)	6 oz	8 oz
5 c food	1# 6 ½ oz (22.5 oz)	7.5 oz	10 oz
6 c food	1# 11 oz (27 oz)	9 oz	12 oz

DOGS

SARDINE AND SALMON ADDITIONS TO DOG MEALS

About sardine and salmon additions to meals

Sardines and wild-caught salmon are an integral part of our program. They provide essential fatty acids and they provide most of the vitamin D that's needed. Sardines and salmon are a relatively low-cost, real food way to provide this essential nutrient. Currently (2013), it seems likely that genetically modified salmon will be approved by the FDA. We recommend making sure that all your ingredients are GMO free.

If you've never fed your dog sardines or salmon, start slowly. This is fat-rich, calorie-dense food. Start by adding a piece of sardine or salmon for a small dog, or a whole sardine for a large dog. If all goes well, with no digestive upsets, increase the amounts.

For animals with any history of a problem with fat, starting slowly is prudent.

You may substitute frozen raw sardines or frozen ground sardines (made by raw pet food companies). Buy canned sardines in water. Sardines packed in oil can be drained, but the oils used are not the best quality and many calories are added to a meal even if the oil is drained. The recipes are computed on drained weight, but you can include the water.

For salmon, we recommend canned products. If you use fresh salmon, always cook it because of the possible parasites it might carry. The bones in fresh cooked salmon must be removed because they're brittle. We have included the bone in fish products in analyzing the diets. Occasional meals including fresh, cooked boneless salmon filets wouldn't upset this balance very much, but if this were always the case the bone meal level would need to be adjusted.

In our meal charts we include the equivalent of one meal of sardines or salmon per week spread over the week by including it with various meat meals – this amount assumes that you feed your animals twice a day.

Including salmon or sardines in dog meals

Sardines are easy to use. The choices that have only water are limited. Although we've used the smaller sardines sometimes with small animals, they are frequently packed in oil. For smaller animals, the extra calories aren't needed, and the oils used aren't the oils we want to add.

For these recipes, we bought examples of the ones that are water packed. Where we live, these included King Oscar, Crown Prince, Brunswick and Chicken of the Sea. Drained weight ranged from 3 – 3.75 ounces. This difference, as with eggs, can add up.

You can also weigh the drained sardines you buy and figure out your proportions using the table that lists proportions by weight.

For salmon, products range from a few ounces to a pound. Divide them up according to the "by weight" table to determine the serving size.

Once you have these serving sizes determined, you can note them on your diet card and never think about it unless you include a new product in your repertoire.

Comparison shopping is advised. At different stores, for the same sardine product, we paid .65 per can or $2.85.

DOGS

BY VOLUME (cups + tablespoons)

DOG	Meat mix + Sardines or Salmon + Veggies		
To make	Meat mix needed	Sardines needed	Veggie mix needed
½ c food	¼ c + ½ T	¼ can	2 T
1 c food	½ c + 1 T	½ can	¼ c
2 c food	1 c + 2 T	1 can	½ c
3 c food	1 ½ c + 3 T	1 ½ cans	¾ c
4 c food	2 ¼ c	2 cans	1 c
5 c food	2 ¾ c + 1 T	2 ½ cans	1 ¼ c
6 c food	3 ¼ + 2 T	3 cans	1 ½ c

BY WEIGHT (ounces + pounds)

DOG	Meat mix + Sardines or Salmon+ Veggies		
To make	Meat mix needed	Sardines needed	Veggie mix needed
½ c food	2.25 oz	.75 oz	1 oz
1 c food	4.5 oz	1.5 oz	2 oz
2 c food	9 oz	3 oz	4 oz
3 c food	13.5 oz	4.5 oz	6 oz
4 c food	1# 2 oz (18 oz)	6 oz	8 oz
5 c food	1# 6 ½ oz (22.5 oz)	7.5 oz	10 oz
6 c food	1# 11 oz (27 oz)	9 oz	12 oz

ESSENTIAL ADDITIONS

Calcium additions for dogs and puppies

The calcium supplement amount in the following tables is not the entire requirement listed by AAFCO for dogs and puppies. It's the requirement minus the amount that's part of the food. The amounts in the tables provide the AAFCO minimum for adult dogs or puppies when combined with food.

Bone meal products range between 20% and 33% calcium. Most bone meal products are acceptable but the serving sizes are different because the percentage of calcium and other minerals differs. It works best for our recipes to narrow that range a little and we've chosen to use products between 24% and 30%. What you see in the serving size columns of each table is what we found in our kitchens with a gram scale and a selection of sensibly shaped measuring spoons. In our kitchens, a level teaspoon weighs about 3 grams. We translated the package directions into grams and then teaspoons for you. We hope one of these choices translates well for you. If you prefer, you can calculate from the table on the opposite page where serving sizes are listed in milligrams. If this is your choice, be sure to look at the calcium amount, not the total bone meal amount.

We've rounded the fractions of teaspoons up or down a bit. For example, since 2.3 grams would be difficult to measure, we're getting as close as we can. There's some room for a bit more of most minerals and total precision isn't possible when preparing home food.

As you can see in the chart, what this may come down to is whether your measuring spoon is rounded or level, - (minus) and + (plus). If you have big animals or lots of them, or you mix up lots of food at a time, it's worth figuring out how much you'd put into 5 or 10 pounds and see how that fits in a measuring cup. Sometimes we do this calculation and add bone meal to a large batch of meat mix.

DOGS

PUPPY (up to about 10 months) BONE MEAL SERVING SIZE

Consult your veterinarian or breeder about when your puppy is mature enough to switch to "dog" status for calcium requirements.

Brand	NOW 30%	KAL 27%	Naturvet 24%
½ c food	½ t -	½ t -	½ t
1 c food	¾ t	¾ t +	1 t +
2 c food	1 ½ t +	1 ¾ t	2 ¼ t
3 c food	2 ½ t -	2 ½ t +	3 ½ t
4 c food	3 ¼ t +	3 ½ t	4 ½ t
5 c food	4 t	4 ½ t	5 ¾ t
6 c food	4 ½ t +	5 ½ t	7 t

DOG BONE MEAL SERVING SIZE

Brand	NOW 30%	KAL 27%	Naturvet 24%
½ c food	¼ t +	¼ t	¼ t
1 c food	½ t -	½ t	½ t
2 c food	¾ t +	1 t scant	1 t
3 c food	1 t	1 ½ t -	2 t
4 c food	1 ¾ t	2 t	2 ½ t
5 c food	2 t +	2 ½ t	3 t
6 c food	2 ½ t	3 t	3 ½ t

Note: Do not use calcium supplements that do not supply phosphorus for puppies or with diets that use high fat ingredients (not our program – we use lean meats). If you have a sick animal that needs phosphorus reduced, that would be an acceptable reason to use a supplement with no phosphorus.

Calcium needs for PUPPIES this recipe rotation only		Calcium needs for DOGS for for this recipe rotation only	
½ cup food	350 mg	½ cup food	195 mg
1 cup food	700 mg	1 cup food	390 mg
1 ½ cup food	1050 mg	1 ½ cup food	585 mg
2 cups food	1400 mg	2 cups food	780 mg
3 cups food	2100 mg	3 cups food	1170 mg
4 cups food	2800 mg	4 cups food	1560 mg
5 cups food	3500 mg	5 cups food	1951 mg
6 cups food	4200 mg	6 cups food	2360 mg

DOGS

Fatty acid additions for dogs

We know that the balance and amount of omega-3 fatty acids is a very important factor in the diets of our animals and ourselves. The level of omega-3 fatty acids needed for any living creature is a controversial topic. Omega-3 fatty acids are very important, but it doesn't take a lot to balance the fatty acids in the diet. There were not huge amounts of DHA and EPA in the ancestral diet.

Common recommendations range up to 1 – 2 teaspoons per 20 pounds of an animal's body weight, and higher for some medical conditions (like cancer). These recommendations for animals often exceed the NRC's safe upper limit, and are frequently many times greater than those recommended for humans. Product serving sizes often recommend the same amount of a fish oil supplement for a 45# dog (1000 kcal per day) as for a human (2000 kcal per day), and this recommendation is on the low end of what we frequently see.

There are reasons not to overdo fatty acid supplements. In people, consuming more than 3 g of fish oil per day can result in increased bleeding, according to an article published in the American Heart Association's "Circulation." Fish oil appears to decrease platelet aggregation, which leads to decreased clotting and prolonged bleeding time. Very large intakes have been associated with hemorrhagic stroke, nosebleeds and blood in urine. Symptoms of omega-3 overdose can include GI symptoms, including reflux, nausea (increased licking and swallowing), vomiting, belching, cramping and diarrhea. MedlinePlus also reports a possible decrease in immune-system activity if high doses of fish oil are taken, resulting in a reduction in the body's ability to fight infection. Probably the most notable symptom of too many omega-3's in animal diets pertains to symptoms of unregulated inflammation. Omega-3's, in proper amounts, control inflammation. If overdone, they enhance the inflammation cascade, resulting in symptoms of inflammation (all of the 'itis' conditions) throughout the body.

There's little basis in science for mega-dosing omega-3 fatty acids. For humans, it seems that more than 500 mg. of a fatty acid product is not effectively used. We don't have that information yet for dogs and cats, but we're all mammals and it's likely that we are similar. From a purely practical point of view, these are really expensive products and there's no reason to give more than can be used. From a functional point of view, megadoses can cause harm given to an animal whose metabololic processes aren't the greatest. If the liver can't break these substances down, and the cells can't use them, then functional problems can result.

Dogs on real food programs that include salmon or sardines need only small amounts of supplementation for fatty acids. Dogs on sub-optimal foods, like dry food, might need more, but amounts still would be less than commonly recommended.

We like krill oil for the phospholipid properties and the astaxanthin content. Krill oils are made by two major manufacturers, and all the brands use one or the other. Levels of EPA and DHA are different. EPA + DHA levels of good fish oils are similar to those of the krill with higher levels. These products are not better or worse, just different.

For ease of use, our chart shows you serving sizes based on the combined amount of EPA and DHA and mg of krill oil. This information is on all labels. Other ways of computing (total omega-3s, capsule size) are confusing and sometimes information is missing. We rounded a bit for the charts with capsules. If one of the choices we give you in the chart works for you, that's the easy choice.

Few fatty acid products have small enough serving sizes to be convenient for daily use. The mercola.com airtight pumpable krill administers 50mg/pump and may be more convenient than puncturing capsules. The table opposite shows how to use capsule products. Liquid fish oils often show 800 – 1200 mg of combined EPA and DHA in one teaspoon. Broken down into serving sizes, a serving my be as little as 1/8 teaspoon per WEEK or 1 capsule per WEEK. You could do this, but we prefer that you spread your fatty acids over more days. You could be less precise and give your tiny dog a drop or two of your capsule and then you take the rest. The Mercola "kid krill" oil product works well for a dog that eats 1 cup of food a day. For this example, one Mercola "kid" capsule a day is the serving size. For larger animals, the oils and larger capsules can be workable but you would probably still be giving this supplement on a weekly basis rather than a daily basis. If that's your choice, plan the supplement for non-fish meal days.

DOGS

For tiny dogs, the quantity needed for oils is so small that the product would certainly be rancid by the time you use it up. If you are using a liquid product for yourself, then it would be appropriate to use it also for your small dog.

All recommendations are based on moderate human recommendations scaled down for dogs and cats. For more concentrated products than the krill oil concentration we suggest, see Table 2.

The following chart shows serving sizes based on the amount of food your dog eats per day, computed according to the calorie count of a cup.

FATTY ACIDS: DAILY SERVINGS FOR DOGS

Table 1	Daily Serving	Krill Oil	Daily Total
cups food	mercola kid or adult krill		approximate desired combined epa + dha
1 c	1 cap Mercola Kid Krill per day	65 – 125 mg	20 mg
2 c	2 caps Mercola Kid krill per day	125 – 150 mg	40 mg
3 c	1 cap Mercola adult	190 – 375 mg	60 mg
4 c	1 cap Mercola adult	250 – 500 mg	75 mg
5 c	1 cap Mercola adult or 1 Neptune	300 – 625 mg	95 mg
6 c	2 caps Mercola adult or 1 Neptune	375 – 750 mg	115 mg

If you choose a concentrated product, it's best to give it on days when you are not already feeding fish, so that you spread out the fatty acids more. Sample liquid fish oils claim up from 800 – 1100 mg combined EPA and DHA per teaspoon on their labels. For capsules, divide over days you are not feeding fish.

As you can see from the chart, for smaller amounts of food it definitely makes more sense to feed a less concentrated product, so you can spread out the serving size over a week.

FATTY ACIDS: WEEKLY SERVINGS FOR DOGS

Table 2	WEEKLY Serving	WEEKLY Serving	WEEKLY Total
cups food	Neptune Krill oil or similar product	Sample fish oil	approximate combined epa + dha desired
1 c	1 cap per week	$^1/_{16}$ – $^1/_8$ t per week	140 mg
2 c	2.25 caps per week	$^1/_8$ – ¼ t per week	280 mg
3 c	3.5 caps per week	¼ – ½ scant t. per week	420
4 c	4.5 caps per week	¼ – ½ scant t. per week	525
5 c	5.5 caps per week	1 scant t per week	665
6 c	6.5 caps per week	1 t per week	800

HOW MUCH DO I FEED MY DOG?

It seems that there should be an easy way to figure out how much food to feed your dog, but there's not. You need to know your dog and you need to develop some skill in evaluating your pet's condition. There are good charts to help you evaluate whether your dog is thin or fat, but breed type, age and other factors make it more complicated than just looking at a chart.

Some dogs are stocky and muscular, with heavy bones. Even thin, they weigh more than lightly boned and muscled dogs of the same general size. A Rottweiler and a Saluki might be the same height, but that's about where the similarities end! Different breeds and breed types have different metabolisms.

Young and old animals may eat different amounts. When your 50-pound Labrador Retriever is six months old, for example, he may eat four pounds of food a day. When he is a mature, active three year old, he might be down to two pounds per day. As an old guy, maybe only one pound.

DOGS

If the Labrador were a Basset Hound of equal weight, his food requirement might decrease sooner than the Labrador. Bassets tend to need less food than many other breeds. A German Shorthair Pointer may burn a lot of food for years, or forever. Pointers can use a lot of calories just keeping warm! Some dogs are built for cold weather and some for hot. Seasonal differences affect how much food your dog needs.

Small dogs burn more food for their size than big dogs and they mature much earlier. Girl dogs of any size tend to start putting on weight at puberty, unlike boy dogs. The effects of spaying and neutering on metabolism are hotly debated. We won't try to cover that topic here, but in general most pets need fewer calories after de-sexing. Clearly, there are many variables and every dog is different.

Puppies may eat twice as much for their size as adults. Learn the growth habits of your breed and your pet's family when it's possible, so you'll have an idea what to expect. For example, one line of Golden Retrievers may be slowing down and maturing at 18 months, while another line is still skinny at three years. Those with no way to obtain family history must rely on observation, but there is much to be learned from body type. If your dog looks like a German Shepherd, he may grow like a German Shepherd. If he's a ten-pound curly mixed-breed, he might grow up fast, like a poodle.

This diet is designed for all life stages. Do not increase any one component for puppies – just feed more food. Feed as much as you need for healthy body condition.

Overweight animals should not lose weight too rapidly. Start out feeding them for slightly under their current weight and adjust so that they lose no more than 1 – 2% of their body weight per month. For example, your Labrador weighs 80 pounds. You're not sure, but you think she should weigh 65 pounds. Figure out how much food she should eat for 75 pounds and feed her that for a week or two. If no weight loss occurs, reduce the amount. Keep reducing as you go. When she gets to 75 pounds, feed her the amount required for 70 pounds. If your dog is obese, enlist assistance from your veterinarian to monitor her health during weight loss and use a 1 – 2% reduction of body weight per month as a goal.

At the other end of the scale, we see dogs that are underweight. They are often performance dogs whose people want them to be as healthy as possible and to them, this means thin. This often happens, too, when dogs are switched to fresh food and start out a bit chubby. Owners get very enthusiastic about their pet's new waistline and just keep going. Ribs and spines should not stick out unless your breed is built that way. Muscular breeds should have muscle. Body fat is needed for many essential functions. Dogs that are too thin cannot build the proper amount of muscle for their body structure. This is an unhealthy state.

If you are switching your overweight dog from dry food to fresh food, it's common to see a significant weight loss in the first week. This is usually the result of the body letting go of water retained due to the inflammatory effects of grain-based food. It's quite impressive, but future weight loss should take place more gradually.

Your food scale will help you keep track of how much you're really feeding. If you always feed your dog one pound of food a day and now he's getting fat or thin, you need to know why, and you need to be sure you know how much you're really giving him.

Is this a seasonal thing? Does he need less food in the summer, more food in the winter, or the reverse? Does he use more calories keeping warm or keeping cool? If you're sure you're giving him the same amount, you can look at exercise, activity and other factors in making sure that all is well. If he's losing weight on the same amount of food, there might be medical trouble brewing — or you might have changed the composition of the food, or conditions have changed. For example, we know one dog who lost several pounds from his 20-pound body when his owner took a three month break from agility training — less exercise for the dog, but no training treats! His owner was afraid he was ill, but when his food level was adjusted, he was fine. On the other hand, weight loss can point to many different health problems, including parasites. Don't ignore unexpected weight loss.

The charts for feeding amounts are given in cups for general guidelines. We show you a range of food amounts that may be appropriate for your pet.

DOGS

The best way to find out what's right for your dog is to start at an appropriate point in the range and see how it goes. Active and young animals start toward the top of the range, and older or chubby animals in the middle. Evaluate your pet's condition frequently! Too much food may cause digestive upset or weight gain. Too little and your dog may become so thin that his body is unable to maintain vital functions.

Directions are based on the calorie count of our recipes. The high end of recommendations in the chart is usually the "official" caloric range. Fresh food veterans agree that animals often maintain weight and condition on ⅓ fewer calories than those recommendations. We've included the entire range of recommendations.

There really are no fast, easy answers. Only experience will show you what's right for your animal.

> **Dog recipes average:**
> **35 calories per ounce,**
> **550 calories per pound.**

Don't get too attached to the categories on the feeding chart. Your individual dog may stay in the food range of a "young/working" dog all his life. Or, he may graduate to the "older/inactive" category when he's two, even though he's pretty active. The amounts are given as a guideline. Each animal is different. "Official" calorie recommendations are based on results with animals eating dry food. In our experience, real food is quite different.

The amount of food that a young, active dog can eat may seem immense, but eventually they grow up and slow down. You need to feed your young growing dog as much as it takes to maintain condition. Do not increase any one component of the diet for young/growing animals. The diet is balanced for all life stages.

Real food, which has all the water still in it, often has less than half the calories of dry food. Our recipe has about 270 calories a cup. A moderate dry food may have more than 500 calories in a cup. You'll get used to the volume of real food.

Unless they are very active, our adult, healthy dogs often maintain good body condition on the amount of food in the "inactive" category. If you calculated the calorie count, it wouldn't seem likely given the charts, but that's our real life experience. Don't assume it will be your experience, but be aware that it's not unusual.

Suggested range of amounts to feed per day

Divide amount by number of meals fed.
Totals are for meat mixed with veggies.

DOG	Puppy	Young/Working	Active Adult	Adult Older/ Inactive
5#	1 ¾ c	1 ¼ c	¾ c	½ c
10#	2 ½ c	2 c	1 ¼ c	1 c
20#	4 – 5 c	3 ½ c	1¾ – 2 c	1 ¼ –1½ c
30#	5 ½ – 7 c	4 ½ – 5 c	2 ⅓ – 2 ¾ c	1 ¾ – 2 c
40#*	6 – 6 ½ c	5 ½ – 6 c	3 – 3 ½ c	2 ¼ – 2 ¾ c
50#*	7 – 8 c	7 c	4 c	3 c
60#*	8 – 9 c	7 – 8 c	4 ½ – 5 c	3 – 4 c
70#*	9 – 10 c	9 c	5 – 5 ½ c	4 c
80#*	9 – 10 c	10 c	6 c	4 ¼ c
90#*	10 ½ c	10 – 11 c	6 ½ c	4 ¾ – 5 c

*We assumed in the puppy column above that few puppies over 40 pounds would be at less than 50% of their adult weight.

For puppies 40 pounds and over, we've given you amounts for pups from 50 – 80% of their adult weight.

For puppies 5 – 30 pounds, amounts are for pups that are at less than 50% of their adult body weight.

DOGS

SUCCESSFUL SWITCHING FOR DOGS

Change your dog over to real food in a way that makes sense to you. It might take a while for you to get comfortable with the whole idea and that's fine. However, your animal's body is probably ready for a new concept in food today and you'll be a hero when you start handing out real food. The total switch can often be accomplished within a week.

If you have been "free feeding," leaving food out all day for your dog, now is a good time to stop. It doesn't entertain them, and it doesn't make up for you being gone. If they get a little hungry while you're gone, that's ok. Dogs aren't built to graze. There's no benefit to this habit and there are many reasons not to do it.

Start by feeding your dog a little bit of fresh food and see how he does with it. If all is well, keep adding a little bit, but start taking out some of his old food. If things are going well, you can usually remove the old food within a few days. Another option is to add the new food as a mid-day snack, to see how he handles it.

If you need to keep feeding some dry food, figure out the appropriate daily amount of fresh food and the daily amount of dry food and use fractions of that daily ration to base your plan on. For example, Rusty eats a cup of dry food a day. You calculate that he would eat a pound of fresh food a day. In the morning, feed him a 1 cup (½ pound) of fresh food (half his daily fresh food ration). In the evening, feed him half of his dry food ration (half a cup). It's best to keep the dry food separate from the fresh, uncooked food. This is just one example. Each individual might be treated differently.

Calculate fresh and dry food separately. Dry food and fresh or canned food have very different calorie counts due to the water in wet foods and the absence of water in dry foods. One cup of dry food has many more calories than one cup of fresh or frozen food, which still contains all the natural water. If you're using commercial foods, you must know the calorie count per pound or ounce so that you can be accurate.

Take this difference into consideration, or you might find yourself seriously underfeeding your dog in the process of switching. We have talked to many people who thought that fresh food was bad for their dog because he lost so much weight. In fact, they were still feeding the one cup a day that was the dog's dry food ration. One cup of dry food could have more than 500 calories. One cup of a moderate-fat meat and veggie diet may have less than 250 calories. When the amount was adjusted and the dogs were fed more, they thrived.

If your pet has loose stools, wait until the stool is firm to continue the transition. If loose stools continue, consult your holistic veterinarian.

You may feed your dog once a day or twice a day. Puppies are fed frequently as babies and less frequently as they mature. Old animals sometimes do better with frequent feedings, as do ill and recovering animals. Otherwise, observe your dog and see what plan you think works best.

There are many medical conditions that are strongly affected by diet. If you want a veterinary opinion that helps you transition your dog to real food, you need to discuss this with a veterinarian who is interested in fresh food diets. Expecting answers that will help you from a dry food supporter is an exercise in frustration, and it will not help your dog.

Many dogs come to real food diets because they have GI problems from diarrhea to Inflammatory Bowel Disease or allergies and hot spots. Dogs with unhealthy guts may not do well on raw food initially. Don't give up! Cook food to start with, and make a transition to raw food over three months. Food can be a miracle cure — but frequently there are bumps in the road and a holistic practitioner can help a lot.

DOGS

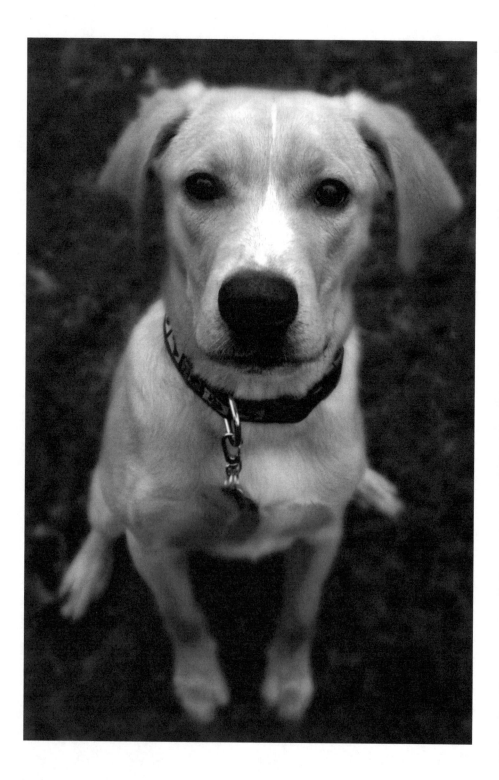

TREATS

WHAT WOULD LIFE BE LIKE WITHOUT TREATS?

There are many excellent commercial meat-based treats. A really good treat costs more per pound than actual food! Sometimes the cost is more than $15.00 per pound even for grocery store choices. In the "natural" pet food aisles, prices shoot toward $30.00 per pound. When reeling from the thought of the increase in cost to feed a pet fresh food, humans often forget that they're paying some seriously steep prices for treats. "Holistic" treats are very expensive. Save them for a special occasion and you might find you have more to spend on food. However, commercial treats are hard to resist, so here are a few guidelines for choosing:

- Read the very, very small print on packages. Some treats are made from ingredients purchased in China or other countries, even though they say "made in the USA." Treats made from US ingredients are less toxic.

- Watch for hidden sources of sugar: cane juice, molasses, honey, brown sugar and fructose are only a few possibilities to exclude from your accept-able choices.

- Buy treats that are made of meat only. Labels are tricky, so learn the language. Meat treats with veggies are available, but often include high-starch ingredients. Read labels carefully.

- Don't buy treats with wheat flour, white flour, oat flour, oats, barley, millet, quinoa or basically any grain ingredients. Some high-carbohydrate treats cause less intestinal havoc than others, but none are necessary or desirable — except they're really cute. Choose the "no gluten" ones and minimize their use.

- We know people with 20 different open bags of treats. They have lots of fun buying them — but with this many open bags, spoilage is an issue. Most treats are best stored in the freezer.

- Cats often vote for freeze-dried nuggets of fish.

Dogs and cats don't care if their treats come out of a cute, expensive package. Meat is pretty popular. So are fruit and small amounts of cheese and other goodies to be found in your refrigerator (raw almonds, cashews, brazil nuts, blueberries, frozen peas — just a few examples!).

"Use small amounts" is a concept that must be learned by most of us. Small for a little dog or a cat would be a ⅛ inch square. Small for a bigger dog might be ⅛ inch to ¼ inch. We love to give treats, but they can add up to enough volume and food value to really unbalance a diet. One way to indulge yourself and your dog is to use all or part of the animal's daily food as treats. This isn't as easy to do with a fresh food diet as with dry food, but it can be done, for at least part of the ration. You can use less meat in your meat and veggie mix and save part of it for treats. You can use your organ meats as treats, making sure that you are including the full amount that's needed (and not a whole lot more). Freeze dried organs are great for this, cut into small pieces. You can use veggies and fruits with low calorie value but high vitamin and antioxidant value - a blueberry or a piece of ripe pepper, or Dr. Becker's favorite treat, frozen peas!

Keep track of what you're handing out for a week or a day to evaluate if you're feeding too many treats. If you're training, you may be feeding more treats than you think. Take a close look at everything you use for treats. You may be handing out some "goodies" that are not very good for your pet. There are countless great choices. For most pets, there's room for occasional indulgence. But in that case, you could share your pizza and forego the carbohydrate-based calorie-rich, expensive "doggie barkery" item.

OPTIMIZING YOUR HOME MADE DIET

We're tempted by the health challenges of our companions to add supplements and herbs. Examine them well. In many cases, our animals have impaired digestion and supplements won't be assimilated until digestive processes are restored and in balance.

"More" is not better

If your pet has "allergies," does it make sense to add an "immune booster" to an already over-reactive system? Probably not. It depends on how that substance acts in the body and on how the body processes it.

If your pet is not digesting food very well (like many with "allergies"), an added substance won't be helpful and may irritate the system. For example, if the liver is already overloaded, perhaps one more substance that is processed by the liver is not a good addition. Existing skin problems caused by an overloaded liver might flare up. Blood values may get worse.

If your pet is in pain and you're thinking of adding a supplement that promises a pain-free life, first remove any pro-inflammatory components in her diet. Grain-based dry food is the primary promoter of inflammation and pain in dogs and cats. Even grain free dry foods contain substantial levels of carbohydrate. You may not need that supplement at all if you eliminate the dietary source of inflammation. It makes better sense to remove a roadblock to health than to feed something that makes your pet feel bad and then give her a supplement (or drug) to take away the pain.

Even if an "expert" has recommended that you use a supplement, ask yourself the following questions:

- "Do I understand how it works in the body?" Will this substance put a burden on an overburdened body? Will it put other nutrients out of proportion? For example, mega-doses of omega-3s may sound great — but in some cases they result in worsening of the symptom they were intended to help.

- "Is it a whole food or an isolated, synthetic substance?" Isolated nutrients don't provide the whole range of nutrients available from a food. In many cases, science has yet to uncover all the relationships, but more and more the conclusion of researchers is "eat whole food."

- "Is it a combination of many "helpful" ingredients?" Sensitive animals and those with impaired digestion are likely to be easily overloaded by "more."

The body takes time to heal. The immune system does not recover all at once. Digestion is complex. It includes not only processing nutrients, but also many critical immune functions. To fulfill all functions, everything has to be working. Be patient with the process.

The supplements below are added to real food to optimize your companion's wellness. You are not required to use any of these additions to balance the diet (with the exception of adding hemp oil to beef food to include needed linoleic acid). We use them all.

We sometimes hear from readers that they're having a hard time finding an ingredient. Everything we suggest is available at good discounts from online vitamin companies. Two that we use frequently are luckyvitamin.com and iherb.com. Supplements may also be found in retail stores like Vitamin Shoppe. Some of the ingredients would indeed be hard to find at your local grocery store.

Optimizing the fat balance in the grocery store chicken, turkey, and beef most of us use for our pet food is not difficult. Grocery store meat does not have the optimal fat profiles found in animals that have been raised naturally, living lives that include food that is their natural diet, normal exercise and access to the outside world.

To improve the fat balance in these meats, we add a little bit of flax oil to the chicken and turkey, or a little bit of hemp oil to the beef.

We don't recommend flax oil as a sole source of omega-3 fatty acids because plant forms of omega-3s aren't well converted to more useful forms of fatty acids such as DHA. We add small amounts to increase the overall level of LA (linoleic acid) and ALA (alpha linoleic acid) and to improve the ratio of these fatty acids so that it resembles that of the ancestral diet in which the short chain omega-6 fatty acid LA (linoleic acid) and the short chain omega-3 fatty acid ALA (alpha linoleic acid) are in a ratio of 2:1 to 6:1.

Our rotation minimizes this problem. However, these oils are an important addition, especially if you must feed one protein source. If you must feed only beef, you MUST include a source of linoleic acid or your diet will be deficient in this nutrient, which is considered essential by the AAFCO. With these oil additions, the amount of LA is adequate for any rotation, and the ratio of LA (linoleic acid, needed for beef) and ALA (alpha linoleic acid) is improved. The overall ratio of omega-6 to omega-3 fatty acids is also improved.

Buy flax and hemp oils in small quantities. Keep them refrigerated. They don't have a long life once opened. If you're using tiny amounts like ½ t a day, you may find that filling a small squeeze bottle with a flip lid helps to get the proper amount into your food and keeps the oil fresher.

For more detailed information on this important topic, see Steve Brown's book, *Unlocking the Canine Ancestral Diet*, available from seespotlivelonger.com.

Cups of food	Chicken/Turkey + flax oil	Beef + hemp oil
½ c	¼ t	¼ t
1 c	½ t	½ t
2 c	1 t	1 t
3 c	1 ½ t	1 ½ t
4 c	2 t	2 t
5 c	2 ½ t	2 ½ t
6 c	2 ¾ t	2 ¾ t

Coconut oil has many benefits to offer. It promotes a healthy balance of organisms in the gut, having antifungal, antibacterial and antiviral properties. It provides medium chain fatty acids which don't require lipase or bile for digestion, so coconut oil is a good way to provide fat for gallbladder and pancreatitis patients. It's easy to digest and assimilate, ideal for sensitive stomachs, IBD, and dysbiosis. Serving size to start with is 1 teaspoon per 10 – 20 pounds per day. Cats are very fond of coconut oil and it's great for them. Keep in mind that fat equals lots of calories so a little might go a long way depending on your pet.

Digestive enzymes are beneficial to all carnivores. There are two parts of a whole prey diet that you'll find are not included in our recipe: fur and guts. Finding fur in your companion's food would be a turn off for most people and feeding entrails is a surefire way to pass parasites up the food chain, which is why you'll not find GI tracts in any raw food recipe. Guts are where most parasites live. In addition there is no pancreas or gall bladder in our recipes. Fur would provide roughage (fiber) and guts (intestines and associated organs and glands) would provide bile, hydrochloric acid, amylase, lipase and protease to enhance digestion. We recommend that you provide digestive enzymes in a more sanitary way: a supplement. There are many to choose from, but they should contain at least a source of amylase (carbohydrate processing enzyme), protease (protein processing enzyme) and lipase (fat processing enzyme). If you can find an enzyme containing bile, as well as betaine (a vegetable source of hydrochloric acid), even better. Enzymes are derived from animal, fungal or vegetable sources. Some pets with allergies can have problems with enzymes derived from fungal sources, so check the label thoroughly. If you're not sure, call the company before you make a purchase. Many human enzyme formulations can be scaled down for pets.

Probiotics are a desirable addition to many diet plans. Probiotics are the beneficial bacterial strains that naturally populate dog and cat GI tracts. We know that animals with a history of gastrointestinal sensitivities, irregularities, and intermittent vomiting and diarrhea benefit from probiotic supplementation. We also know that recent research demonstrates that animals fighting cancer, auto-immune disease, organ degeneration and detoxification challenges benefit from probiotic supplementation. Human probiotic strains have been formulated to repopulate human GI flora. Dogs and cats have a different population of normal flora. Giving human probiotics (lactobacillus/bifidus/acidophilus) can provide some benefit. Providing additional species-appropriate bacterial strains (E. faecalis, etc.) can be more beneficial. At mercola.com you will find a product designed specifically for dogs and cats.

Because "probiotics" are currently trendy there are a lot of products on the market. Many human and pet probiotics are a worthless investment of money in terms of viable, transferrable Colony Forming Units (CFU's). Make sure you do your research and trust the company you are purchasing from.

Super green foods are foods packed with an above-average dose of naturally occurring phytonutrients, antioxidants, essential fatty acids, vitamins and minerals. Wheatgrass, chlorella, dulse, blue-green algae (AFA), barleygrass, spirulina, astaxanthin, kelp and alfalfa are a few of the superfoods that can provide additional health benefits above and beyond a balanced meat and veggie diet.

Don't get in a rut with these great foods. In our previous version we advised against the use of kelp and alfalfa. This was because we've known many animals that developed allergies to these fine foods by eating them every day. Also, many people use plain kelp for their pet's iodine requirements – this is not a reliable way to be sure your pet is getting the proper amount of iodine. Use a standardized kelp product for this purpose, not a bucket of kelp that you get at a pet store.

From helping to speed wound healing to fighting cancer, super green food supplements can benefit almost every pet. We recommend rotating through them all, switching products every time you run out to avoid any allergic reactions as well as allowing your pet to receive the nutritional benefits from all of these miracle foods.

Doses vary, depending on the product. Scale down from the human recommendations on the bottle (if a human dose is 2 tablespoons daily, a 75 lb dog would be about 1 tablespoon, and a 40 lb dog would be about 1 ½ teaspoons a day, etc.). For dogs, it would be nearly impossible to overdose on green foods, so don't panic about exact measurement.

For cats, you could add too much and end up with a urinary pH that is high enough to cause trouble. If you stick to a "pinch" for a cat, there will be no problem. A pinch is a literal pinch – what you can pick up between two fingers. We especially love green foods if your pets don't have access to chlorophyll naturally (in the form of pesticide-free grass to graze on).

Fiber was discussed in the general additions section, to be added if your pet seems to need more fiber if she has trouble defecating or if she has very dry stools.

A glandular supplement is a powder made up of the tiny glands and organs that we are not able to supply to our animals. These organs and glands are components of the natural diet that are missing in almost all diets. They include (in addition to the heart and liver we are able to provide) pituitary, hypothalamus, adrenal, pancreas, spleen and other substances. Thyroid hormone is classified as a drug, so if a glandular product includes thyroid, the hormone has been removed. Glandular products are available in capsule and powder form to be added to food. There are many human glandular products, but most have a specific purpose. What you're looking for is a formula for general support.

We include heart and liver in planning a diet – they're fairly easy to find. The other parts of a whole prey animal are beyond our reach (unless you become truly dedicated). To support organ systems and the function of the whole body, it may be of great benefit to include a glandular product. Check mypetsfriend.com for glandular products (Pet G.O.) for your pet. These products are reasonably priced but not usually found in pet stores. For this product, you might have to buy online. We hope to have our own product soon.

Joint support in the form of supplemental chondroprotective agents is beneficial for many pets. These are specific supplements that nourish and rebuild cartilage. By offering your pet joint support during the aging process you can slow the degenerative changes in the joints.

Glucosamine sulfate stimulates the production of proteoglycans and collagen that can strengthen your pet's articular cartilage. Chondroitin sulfate also strengthens cartilage, making your pet's joints more resilient against the effects of arthritis. Additionally, chondroitin sulfate has been shown to be effective in inhibiting destructive enzymes that break down articular cartilage. MSM (methylsulfonylmethane) supplies bio-available sulphur that is a key nutrient in the synthesis of collagen, the growth and repair of connective tissues and maintenance of joint fluid, among a variety of other biologic functions. All three of these substances are naturally found in your pet's body, but the body's ability to produce adequate amounts decreases with age as well as joint trauma or stress.

Dose suggestions for joint support:

- 10 mg per lb daily for maintenance/wellness
- 20 mg per lb 1-2 times daily for therapeutic serving to slow degenerative musculoskeletal changes

Milk thistle protects liver cells from toxic insults from a variety of sources: heartworm medications, flea/tick insecticides, mercury and heavy metals, lawn and garden herbicides and the effects of anesthesia. You should discuss what dose is right for your pet for each particular situation. Pertaining to heartworm medication detoxification, we recommend giving dogs milk thistle daily for **one week** after each heartworm pill to assist in detoxification. Most standardized milk thistle capsules are 100 – 125 mg.

Dose suggestions:

- small dogs and cats ½ capsule daily
- medium dogs 1 capsule daily
- large/giant dogs 1 capsule twice daily

Ubiquinol (the more absorbable form of CoQ10) has a critical role in producing cellular energy, or ATP (adenosine triphosphate). This is the energy used to fuel your pet's entire body. Supplementation has been proven to be beneficial in fighting gum disease, high blood pressure, heart, kidney, eye, neurologic and respiratory diseases. It is an excellent supplement for all pets. Daily doses range from 1 – 5 mg per lb. per day.

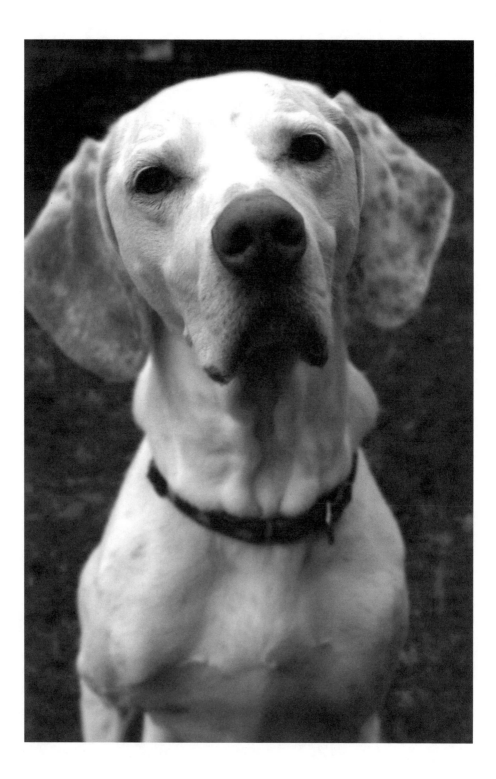

COMMERCIAL FROZEN FOODS

Commercial fresh frozen diets and the stores and websites that specialize in healthier options for pets have multiplied and thrived in recent years. The products available have become more than an oddball special order item. Freezers filled with raw pet food are found even in big chain stores. These products can be very good and they can help you out when there's just not time to make food.

It's necessary to know your way around these products. Retail personnel are usually dedicated and concerned, but they don't always really know about the nutritional makeup of the foods. You need to know the calorie content, the amount of veggies and the fat/protein/carbohydrate amounts in order to compare.

There are two categories of commercial frozen foods. Complete diets are formulated to meet the AAFCO guidelines for all life stages. Component products are designed to allow you to put together your own diet.

Component products are useful for providing more protein sources than are commonly available, and they often have frozen and freeze dried organ meats as part of the line. As long as you're aware that these are not complete diets, they can be great additions to your plan.

Complete products have a very wide range of nutrition profiles. If you're under-informed, you can get into trouble. The labels may say they are "complete" but the numbers may disagree.

The inclusion of vegetables affects the nutrition profile considerably because veggies take up space but don't have a lot of calories. A low veggie 8-ounce patty might have 600 – 700 calories. 8 ounces of a higher veggie food might have 300 calories. (Sales people may tell you that you're just paying for water in a higher veggie food. In fact, that water holds valuable nutrients.)

These differences can make a scary change in an animal in a very short time. Fast and dangerous weight loss can occur, and just as swift weight gain, even if you follow the guidelines of the manufacturer or the store salesperson. A high fat diet fed to an animal whose digestive system is not in excellent shape (you may not know this) can lead to pancreatitis, which can be painful and even fatal.

Use caution when following feeding directions for commercial products. Recommendations are often made for very different products, which may not be immediately clear. For example, one brand sells both canned and raw frozen food, two products that seem similar. You might think that these could be substituted equally, but it's recommended that customers feed their pets twice the amount of canned food as raw food. In this case, the canned food has more water in it than the raw frozen food. The canned food has fewer calories per cup. If you fed your pet canned food according to the frozen directions, your dog would lose weight at an alarming rate. Read carefully and thoroughly! Directions are only a guideline.

To be close to the ancestral diet, a food should have about half as much fat as protein. For example, a food that is 12% protein as fed should be about 6% or 5% fat. Otherwise, many more fat calories are provided than protein. Since fat has more than twice as many calories as protein, it can easily displace protein in the diet, and you're quickly feeding your dog or cat a balance overwhelmingly on the fat side — often as much as 75 – 80% of the calories are fat. This is common in the diets that have almost no vegetables, but even in the higher veggie foods some varieties and brands may have high levels of fat. Fat is cheap and it makes the portion size smaller — and thus it can be cheaper to feed a higher fat food, but it's not the best choice unless your animals are active athletes who burn off the calories in healthy ways.

It's common for foods to list fat percentages close to 6%, but the calorie statement may not agree with this percentage. Brand 3 in the table lists 6% fat and 1040 calories per pound. At 1040 calories per pound, that food is probably 18% fat, which means that more than 70% of the calories come from fat. If it were really 6%, about 46% of the calories would come from fat – very close to the ancestral level. Steve Brown, who consults for many fresh food diet companies, says that the most accurate number in this situation is likely to be the calorie count.

Using caloric information to determine probable fat content
(from company websites)

	Ancestral	Brand 1	Brand 2	Brand 3
calories per # from website		500 kcal	695	1040
fat % on label	6%	4%	9%	6%
probable actual fat %		6%	9%	18%
% of dietary calories from fat	46%	46%	53%	72%

Note: Atwater factors used in all calculations

The easiest way to compare without complicated calculations is just to go by the calorie count given on the label. If it is much above our recipe (about 35 – 40 kcal per ounce, 550 – 650 kcal per pound), you are buying a product that is higher in fat and calories than our recipe. You'll have to reduce the amount of food you feed, and you won't be feeding a nutrition profile that is similar to the ancestral diet.

We like to use the moderate products. For dogs, the ones that include 20% – 30% veggies and fruits by volume are the closest to our plan and to their evolutionary diet. For cats, the lower to very low veggie foods are appropriate, but cats should also have appropriate fat content, a bit less than half the protein level given on the label. Low-veggie commercial products often have very high fat content.

We hear from frustrated people who can't find a food that meets these guidelines in the freezer in their local store. We're sorry, and we hope that manufacturers find ways to come closer to ancestral profiles. Fortunately, there are some products that do have appropriate levels of protein and fat.

In canned foods, the calorie difference is often related to water – foods with fewer calories have more water. In frozen foods, this might be true too, but the difference can be that there are more veggies – which have more water proportionately to their food value.

There are many choices, whether for foods to be shipped direct to your door or bought in a store. Choose what comes closest to our lean diet goal, and what agrees with your pet best.

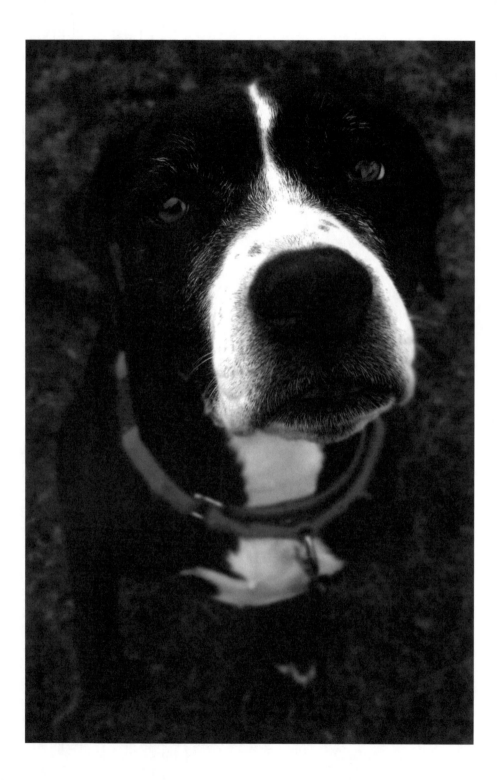

FOOD FOR A LIFETIME

Maybe you started making food for your dog or cat because you want to maintain perfect health and you want to extend the good food program you follow to your pet. You learned about fresh food and decided that you have room in your life for the tasks involved in the process. If so, you're a hero. Most of us began making food because we had a sick dog or cat. Fresh food was one of the main factors in returning our animals to health. We're grateful!

But do you really have to keep doing this forever? Wouldn't your dog be fine if you fed him good dry food again? After all, the problems that brought you to making your own food are fixed, aren't they? Perhaps you sometimes find yourself grinding your teeth as you look in the freezer and see that once again, the food is almost gone… time to do it all over again.

The basic questions are:

- Do I really have to do this?
- When can I go back to dry food?

The answers:

- Yes, you need to feed fresh food.
- You can't go back to dry food if you want to keep the gains you've made.

The answer is simple. Real food is best.

The reason your pet is healthy now is that you feed him fresh food. If you had a sick animal, and he's better now, going back to dry food will bring back the problem — which was probably caused by nutrition originally. If you have been so successful that the entire problem is healed, give thanks.

Nutrition-induced conditions are often functional, not medical – though you may have spent thousands of dollars with veterinarians figuring out what's wrong. If you provide good food, fresh air, exercise and lots of love many conditions improve or heal themselves.

If you go back to the dry food routine that most of us started out with, your animal might be fine temporarily. But you should not be surprised to see old symptoms return eventually. Now that you know more than you did about how the body works you know that we can't always fix things that go wrong.

Years later you could be faced with disease that progresses fast enough that diet change is no longer a simple solution.

If you just can't fit food preparation into your life, investigate commercial products. Make use of them and make your own food when you can.

There may be times when you must supplement with dry food for economic reasons, or just due to the fluctuations of life. Be kind to yourself. Do the best you can and get back to healthier food as soon as it's workable in your life.

One more thing…

We think that food is really important. That's pretty obvious.

Just as important is fitness. Every cell in the body needs to be fit to function. For everything to function, from organs to circulation to guts to cells, everything must get a chance to work. The best food in the world won't be able to do its job if the being who eats the food has a life that consists of sleeping on the couch between meals. Enjoy yourself and your animals! Get outside with your dogs and play with your cats – real exercise is one of the foundations of health.

When people start to learn about tools for healthier living for their animals, they find their lives changed in many ways.

It's possible to find a way to feed a meat-based, species-appropriate diet in almost any household, whether your tastes run to intensive or minimal preparation. The benefits of improving diet, however, extend far beyond the actual food.

Our lives are immeasurably enriched when we take the time to be involved in the process of living. We appreciate the miraculous world around us more and we become far better connected to our animals and each other.

We hope you find this to be true for yourself and all the animals who touch your life.

A HOMEMADE MINERAL/VITAMIN MIX

"You can trace every sickness, every disease, every ailment to mineral deficiency"

two time Nobel Prize winner Linus Pauling

Our 3rd edition has some recipe revisions that reduce the amount of supplementation needed. For example, with liver amounts increased a bit, no copper is needed for cats or dogs in our rotation. We chose to use the lower NRC guidelines instead of AAFCO for zinc. The result of our revision is that our supplement recipes have fewer ingredients and lower quantities of some ingredients.

The minerals needed are often small quantities, and the serving size for one animal may be tiny. If you get a little bit too much, it's not going to be a problem. The range between what's needed according to the standards, what was probably in the ancestral diet, and what might be toxic is huge. Buy simple metal measuring spoons and you should be fine.

We are including two recipes for cats and two recipes for dogs. In our rotation we tried to get as close as we could to providing all nutrients from food alone, and recipe A provides the few missing pieces. We think those of you who share this goal want to add as little in the way of supplementation as possible. If you're feeding a good rotation and including eggs, organs, and sardines or salmon, use recipe A. You'll see that no copper supplementation is needed for either cats or dogs, no vitamin D is needed, and quantities needed of other nutrients may be lower because these nutrients are coming from food.

Recipe B provides for situations that might have some deficits. If you're just getting started and you haven't got all the pieces quite integrated, or your cat refuses to eat eggs, or you have to feed just beef temporarily, or if you are experiencing any of the myriad "diet in process" glitches that might arise, use recipe B.

Serving sizes are not a lot different between recipes, but ingredients are, so use the proper recipe for your situation.

Salt is low in a homemade diet. We've been told that salt is bad for us, but salt is essential in maintaining the electrical balance of the body and for many critical biological and cellular functions. In the natural diet, part of the salt would come from blood and spleen and organs we don't feed. Plain salt is the base for our mineral/vitamin recipe.

Iron is a trace mineral needed to make hemoglobin, the protein needed to carry oxygen throughout the body. Hemoglobin gives red blood cells their color, and stores most of the body's iron supply. Iron is also stored in muscle tissue, and helps supply the muscles with the oxygen needed to make them work normally.

We used NOW® 18 mg Chelated Iron Biglycinate capsules.

Copper is necessary for a number of body processes including the formation of collagen, bone and connective tissue, the absorption of iron, the development and maturation of red blood cells, and the development of pigment in hair.

Some canine breeds have a genetic problem with copper. In the main rotation no supplementation is needed. If you have a breed with this problem, you can leave the copper out of recipe B and it will not affect serving size much.

We used Twinlabs® Chelated Copper 2 mg capsules. Copper is often sold in combination with zinc, but the balance is not appropriate. Purchase these minerals separately.

Manganese is important for normal thyroid function, blood sugar control, and normal skeletal growth. Manganese is essential for a healthy metabolism, reproduction, and the action of many enzymes in the body responsible for the production of energy and making fatty acids.

We used Twinlabs® 10 mg Chelated Manganese capsules.

Zinc is needed in every single cell. Your pet's body needs zinc for structural and energy producing functions. Zinc is critical for the production of protein, and it's a trigger for many biochemical reactions, including the production of DNA. Zinc is necessary for the production and activation of T-cells, a type of white blood cell that is involved in battling infections. Zinc empowers the immune system to fight disease. It is also a critical nutrient for healthy skin. We have used the NRC standards for zinc.

Some individuals in some breeds have difficulty assimilating zinc. If it is recommended that your animals receive more than the normal level of zinc, add the extra amount to the food, not to the supplement recipe. Additions to the supplement recipe would change the weight and serving size.

We used NOW® 50 mg Zinc Picolinate capsules.

Iodine is critical for normal growth and development. Iodine is needed for adequate thyroid gland hormone production. Thyroid hormones control the basic metabolic rate of the body, facilitate optimal utilization of calories and are required for other glandular (endocrine) balances.

Iodine from kelp is easy to find, but you must buy a product that's standardized, not just dry kelp. In dry kelp products, iodine content can vary enough so that you might not have enough – or too much.

We used NOW® Kelp with iodine standardized to 150 mcg iodine per tablet.

Vitamin D is plentiful in a diet with sardines and wild salmon. Organ meats provide some vitamin D, but without the salmon and sardine components to your diet program, vitamin D would not be adequate. The available data on vitamin D is sparse and unreliable currently, so we include enough in supplement recipe B to cover any deficits.

We used Twinlabs 400 iu "dry" vitamin D.

Vitamin E is very slightly deficient. We used "dry" E 400 iu tablets made by Solgar or Twin Labs.

Folic acid is slightly deficient for cats according to AAFCO standards. This slight shortfall is covered in the cat recipes.

We used NOW® Folic Acid 800 mcg with B12.

Taurine is considered an essential nutrient for cats by AAFCO. We think it's highly likely that taurine is needed by all living creatures. Taurine is easily damaged and lost in processing. Data for taurine is difficult to find and not very reliable, so we are including it in recipes to make sure there's enough.

We used NOW® Taurine 1 gram capsules.

Choline is an essential nutrient with a high requirement for cats compared to dogs and humans. It is abundant in organ meats and eggs, and present in other meats, vegetables, and fruits. In a full rotation that includes organ meats and eggs, this requirement is met. For cats, however, in a restricted diet there are shortages from 75-175 mg per pound of food. Supplements to supply this deficiency are not easy to use: they can't be added to the mineral/vitamin mix to cover potential deficits, as we have done for other nutrients. Granular lecithin is one choice, but it's not likely to have many fans among cats. ½ – 1 teaspoon would be needed per cup of food. One possibility is Phosphatidyl Choline capsules, available at health food stores. We prefer that you feed organ meats and eggs!

The recipes make enough vitamin/mineral supplement for 50# of food. The products we used are easy to find online or in a full-service health food store.

To calculate the supplement, we multiplied nutrition needs per pound of food by 50. We divided that according to the grams, milligrams, or micrograms provided by the supplements to get the number of capsules needed per recipe, weighed the results and computed the serving size from that result.

The foundation of the supplement is salt, which is needed in the basic diet. We analyzed the recipes with the salt listed in these supplements included, so you will not be adding more salt to the recipe than shows on the analyses. There are a few medical conditions in which it might be advisable to limit salt, in which case you could use an equal volume of some inert substance and come out with the same serving size.

We counted out the ingredients and ground them in a coffee grinder (or blender) until very fine. We weighed the resulting powder and divided by 50 to get the weight of a serving for one pound of food and then divided or multiplied to get serving sizes for smaller or larger amounts.

If you choose to make your own recipe based on the charts for individual meat versions of a fresh food diet (analyses follow in the next appendix), follow this process. You would need a gram scale.

As discussed earlier in this book, measuring spoons vary radically. Simple metal measuring spoons provide the most consistent amounts but even within those, measurements may differ. Cute measuring spoons that look like oranges or tomatoes (just one example of many) are not likely to be accurate, especially in the smaller sizes. If you're measuring small quantities, we've concluded it's better to just use ⅛ or ¼ teaspoons and estimate a half of that amount than to buy the tiny ones – which are just as inconsistent as the fancy ceramic ones.

CAT SUPPLEMENT RECIPE A

Recipe for a program that includes all components, with organs, eggs and sardines or salmon

CAT supplement recipe A for 50# of food

Salt	20 g (1 level tablespoon)	
	CAPSULES OR TABLETS	TOTAL MG NEEDED
Iron	9	162 mg
Manganese	3	30 mg
Iodine (from standardized kelp)	3	450 mcg
Folic acid	3	240 mcg
Vit E	3	120 iu
Taurine	25	25 grams

Number or capsules or tablets recommended is based on the brand we suggested.

CAT supplement A serving sizes

AMOUNT OF FOOD	SUPPLEMENT SERVING SIZE
½ cup	⅛ t scant (half a 1/8 t measure)
1 cup	⅛ t
2 cups	¼ t

Count out all your ingredients and grind them in a coffee grinder or a blender with the lid shut tight. There's no need to empty the capsules, just grind them all up. This is a dusty process. Let the contents settle for a bit before you open the lid.

- Stir your vitamin/mineral mix every time you use it. Contents can settle over time.
- Store in a glass jar that has a tight lid.
- Make sure your measuring spoon is dry so moisture doesn't contaminate the mix.

CAT SUPPLEMENT RECIPE B

For programs that may have deficits

CAT supplement recipe B for 50# of food

Salt	20 g (1 level tablespoon)	
	CAPSULES OR TABLETS	TOTAL MG NEEDED
Iron	25	450 mg
Copper	15	30 mg
Manganese	5	50 mg
Zinc	7	350 mg
Iodine (from standardized kelp)	20	3000 mcg
Vitamin D	15	6000 iu
Folic acid	6	4800 mcg
Vit E	3	120 iu
Taurine	25	25 grams

Number or capsules or tablets recommended is based on the brand we suggested.

CAT supplement B serving sizes

AMOUNT OF FOOD	SUPPLEMENT SERVING SIZE
½ cup	⅛ t -
1 cup	⅛ t +
2 cups	¼ t +

Count out all your ingredients and grind them in a coffee grinder or a blender with the lid shut tight. There's no need to empty the capsules, just grind them all up. This is a dusty process. Let the contents settle for a bit before you open the lid.

- Stir your vitamin/mineral mix every time you use it. Contents can settle over time.

- Store in a glass jar that has a tight lid.

- Make sure your measuring spoon is dry so moisture doesn't contaminate the mix.

DOG SUPPLEMENT RECIPE A

Recipe for a program that includes all components, with organs, eggs and sardines or salmon

DOG supplement recipe A for 50# of food

Salt	25 g (4 teaspoons)	
	CAPSULES OR TABLETS	TOTAL MG NEEDED
Iron	13	234 mg
Manganese	2	20 mg
Zinc	5	250 mg
Iodine (from standardized kelp)	65	9.75 mg
Vitamin E	3	1200 iu
Taurine	25	25 grams

Number or capsules or tablets recommended is based on the brand we suggested.

DOG supplement A serving sizes

AMOUNT OF FOOD	SUPPLEMENT SERVING SIZE
½ cup	⅛ t -
1 cup	¼ t -
2 cups	½ t -
3 cups	½ t +
4 cups	¾ t +
5 cups	1 t
6 cups	1 ¼ t

Count out all your ingredients and grind them in a coffee grinder or a blender with the lid shut tight. There's no need to empty the capsules, just grind them all up. This is a dusty process. Let the contents settle for a bit before you open the lid.

- Stir your vitamin/mineral mix every time you use it. Contents can settle over time.

- Store in a glass jar that has a tight lid.

- Make sure your measuring spoon is dry so moisture doesn't contaminate the mix.

DOG SUPPLEMENT RECIPE B

For programs that may have deficits

DOG supplement recipe B for 50# of food

Salt	25 g (4 teaspoons)	
	CAPSULES OR TABLETS	TOTAL MG NEEDED
Iron	16	288
Copper	19	38
Manganese	3	30
Zinc	9	450
Iodine (from standardized kelp)	75	11.25
Vitamin D	8	3200 iu
Vitamin E	3	1200 iu
Taurine	25	25 grams

Number or capsules or tablets recommended is based on the brand we suggested.

DOG supplement B serving sizes

AMOUNT OF FOOD	SUPPLEMENT SERVING SIZE
½ cup	⅛ t
1 cup	¼ t
2 cups	½ t
3 cups	¾ t rounded
4 cups	1 t
5 cups	1 ¼ t
6 cups	1 ½ t

Count out all your ingredients and grind them in a coffee grinder or a blender with the lid shut tight. There's no need to empty the capsules, just grind them all up. This is a dusty process. Let the contents settle for a bit before you open the lid.

- Stir your vitamin/mineral mix every time you use it. Contents can settle over time.

- Store in a glass jar that has a tight lid.

- Make sure your measuring spoon is dry so moisture doesn't contaminate the mix.

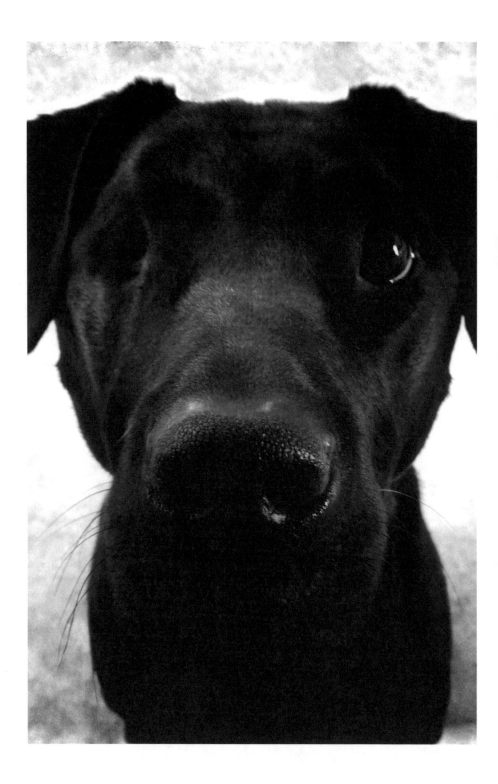

APPENDIX II – ANALYSIS OF INDIVIDUAL DIETS

This appendix shows you the nutrient breakdown of different versions of our rotation. Our goal with this program was to provide a home-prepared, meat and vegetable based diet that meets nutrition needs for all life stages. Our premise is that with some planning and a little attention to detail, we should be able to accomplish this goal using mostly whole foods, without major supplementation or use of ingredients that are difficult to find.

As you can see from the analysis of the complete rotations, it is indeed possible to get very close to meeting nutrition needs with a simple, well planned diet of fresh foods in a species-appropriate balance.

For rotation analyses (except the two including ground bone) we include the bone meal needed for proper calcium/phosphorus balance, the salt that is the base of the supplement, and the amount of krill oil we suggest. For analyses of one-protein recipes, we took these ingredients out to show the bare bones of the recipe.

In order to avoid information overload, we are showing you this information per pound of food, instead of including "per 1000 kcal," which is how the original analysis is done. Those who use this information are feeding real animals, not just comparing data, so we gave you the charts with the information on each analysis calculated down from "per 1000 kcal" to "per pound," which is 2 cups of food.

When a chart says "DOG" or "CAT" we are referring to the species – all recipes are formulated to be appropriate for all life stages. For example, this means that the column "AAFCO requirement" will be a percentage of the AAFCO requirement per 1000 kcal (or NRC requirement in some cases).

You may notice that the numbers in the column "AAFCO requirement per pound" differ somewhat. This is because different versions vary in their calorie count, and each calculation is done using the calorie count of that specific version.

Also notice that the amounts may be g (grams), mg (milligrams), or IU (international units). This can get confusing when you try to buy a supplement that's sold in mcg (micrograms) but the chart says mg (milligrams). Be careful with your decimal points and you'll be ok. We used the measurements in the chart because they correspond to the measurements used by AAFCO and NRC.

We used NRC recommendations for zinc. We used the AAFCO copper requirement for cats for canned food. NRC has begun to establish wider recommendations for fatty acids, so we used those recommendations.

Iodine is a very important nutrient that is not just in short supply but that is almost absent from most home-prepared diets. Other minerals may be at a lower level than is probably optimal without supplementation, but with NO iodine, we can be sure that over time there will be a problem. Very few foods supply iodine, and we must supplement this important nutrient. Our supplement recipe provides iodine. If you choose to make your own supplement, you have more flexibility in the form you choose to use. Just be very sure that you include it.

This collection of analyses (each for dog or cat) includes the versions we think will be most useful and needed.

- Some readers may wish to make their own nutrient supplement recipes. Using the information on these charts, it's possible to do so.
- There are two basic charts: the complete rotation with bone meal, and the complete rotation if you use the meat with bone versions.
- The third basic chart shows you the improvement in the rotation if you add flax and hemp to the complete rotation. If you are feeding grass-fed and finished beef and pasture raised poultry, you wouldn't need to consider these additions, but they are useful for those using grocery store meats.
- There may be reasons to feed only one protein. We show you chicken, beef, and turkey alone. These recipes are analyzed without salt.
- Some animals may refuse to eat fish or eggs, so we show you how these omissions affect the outcome.
- And then there are those of us who just like to know.

(Recipes average 500 kcal (dog) and 600 kcal (cat) per pound, so if you want to know approximate kcal per 1000 kcal, you can calculate using percentages based on those numbers.)

CAT Chicken, turkey, beef, organs, eggs, sardines and veggies with bone meal + krill

MACRONUTRIENTS	As fed	% of calories	DM
Protein	16%	49%	62%
Fat	7%	48%	27%
Moisture	74%		0%
Ash	2%		7%
Carbohydrate	0.8%	3%	4%

MICRONUTRIENTS	Additional nutrients needed per pound	Nutrient per pound of this recipe	AAFCO requirement per pound this recipe
Calcium, g		1.63	1.48
Phosphorus, g		1.28	1.18
Calcium/Phosphorus Ratio	1.3: 1		
Potassium, g		1.16	0.89
Sodium, g		0.33	0.30
Magnesium, g		0.11	0.12
Iron, mg	3.30	8.53	11.82
Copper, mg		0.80	0.74
Manganese, mg	0.53	0.29	1.12
Zinc, mg (NRC)		10.90	10.95 (NRC)
Iodine, mg	.01	0.04	0.05
Selenium, mg		0.10	0.02

VITAMINS			
Vit A IU		6023.00	1,331.00
Vit D IU		173.00	111.23
Vit E IU		6.96	4.44
Thiamine mg	0.40	0.33	0.74
Riboflavin mg		1.29	0.59
Pantothenic Acid mg		4.97	0.74
Niacin mg		19.93	8.88
B6 (Pyridoxine) mg		1.43	0.59
Folic acid mg	0.04	0.07	0.12
Biotin mg			0.013
Vit B12 mg		0.009	0.0029
Choline mg		360.00	360.00
Taurine g	–	–	0.30

FATS	Amount in 1 pound of this recipe	Recommended per pound NRC
LA g	4.73	0.84
ALA g	0.30	0.03
AA g	0.42	0.03
EPA + DHA combined	0.53 g (EPA .20, DHA .33)	0.015 g
Overall omega-6/omega-3 ratio: 5.9: 1		600 kcal per pound

CAT Chicken, turkey, beef, organs, eggs, sardines and veggies with bone meal, krill, flax, + hemp

MACRONUTRIENTS	As fed	% of calories	DM
Protein	16%	47%	60%
Fat	8%	50%	29%
Moisture	74%		0%
Ash	1.9%		7%
Carbohydrate	0.9%	3%	3%

MICRONUTRIENTS	Additional nutrients needed per pound	Nutrient per pound of this recipe	AAFCO requirement per pound this recipe
Calcium, g		1.62	1.53
Phosphorus, g		1.27	1.22
Calcium/Phosphorus Ratio	1.3: 1		
Potassium, g		1.16	0.92
Sodium, g		0.33	0.31
Magnesium, g		0.11	0.12
Iron, mg	4.00	8.47	12.25
Copper, mg		0.79	0.77
Manganese, mg	0.87	0.29	1.16
Zinc, mg (NRC)	0.53	10.81	11.33 (NRC)
Iodine, mg	0.01	0.044	0.055
Selenium, mg		0.10	0.02

VITAMINS			
Vit A IU		5986.00	1,380.00
Vit D IU		172.67	115.00
Vit E IU		8.30	4.60
Thiamine mg	0.44	0.32	0.77
Riboflavin mg		1.28	0.61
Pantothenic Acid mg		4.94	0.77
Niacin mg		19.80	9.20
B6 (Pyridoxine) mg		1.42	0.61
Folic acid mg	0.05	0.07	0.12
Biotin mg	–	–	0.013
Vit B12 mg		0.009	0.0031
Choline mg	26.74	341.00	367.00
Taurine g	–	–	0.31

FATS	Amount in 1 pound of this recipe	Recommended per pound NRC
LA g	5.50	0.84
ALA g	1.20	0.03
AA	0.40	0.03
EPA + DHA combined	0.52 g (EPA .2, DHA .32)	0.015 g
Overall omega-6/omega-3 ratio: 3:1		610 kcal pr pound

CAT Chicken, turkey, beef, organs, eggs, sardines and veggies with ground bone + krill

MACRONUTRIENTS	As fed	% of calories	DM
Protein	16%	54%	65%
Fat	6%	42%	23%
Moisture	75%		0%
Ash	1.8%		7%
Carbohydrate	1.1%	4%	4%

MICRONUTRIENTS	Additional nutrients needed per pound	Nutrient per pound of this recipe	AAFCO requirement per pound this recipe
Calcium, g		1.76	1.35
Phosphorus, g		1.42	1.08
Calcium Phosphorus Ratio	1.25: 1		
Potassium, g		1.19	0.81
Sodium, g		0.37	0.27
Magnesium, g		0.16	0.11
Iron, mg	2.32	8.49	10.82
Copper, mg		1.63	0.68
Manganese, mg	0.70	0.33	1.03
Zinc, mg (NRC)		12.23	10.95 (NRC)
Iodine, mg	0.01	0.04	0.05
Selenium, mg		0.09	0.02

VITAMINS			
Vit A IU		9138.00	1,216.94
Vit D IU		170.00	102.00
Vit E IU		6.62	4.00
Thiamine mg	0.36	0.32	0.68
Riboflavin mg		1.48	0.54
Pantothenic Acid mg		5.13	0.68
Niacin mg		17.69	8.13
B6 (Pyridoxine) mg		1.38	0.54
Folic acid mg		0.10	0.11
Biotin mg	–	–	0.013
Vit B12 mg		0.02	0.0029
Choline mg		355.00	324.00
Taurine g	–	–	0.27

FATS	Amount in 1 pound of this recipe	Recommended per pound NRC
LA g	2.66	0.84
ALA g	0.17	0.03
AA g	0.59	0.03
EPA + DHA combined	0.58 g (EPA .21, DHA .37)	0.0135 g
Overall omega-6/omega-3 ratio: 4: 1		542 kcal per pound

CAT Chicken, turkey, beef and veggies with bone meal + krill: NO Eggs, NO Sardines, NO Organs

MACRONUTRIENTS	As fed	% of calories	DM
Protein	16%	48%	61%
Fat	8%	51%	29%
Moisture	74%		0%
Ash	1.8%		7%
Carbohydrate	0.5%	2%	2%

MICRONUTRIENTS	Additional nutrients needed per pound	Nutrient per pound of this recipe	AAFCO requirement per pound this recipe
Calcium, g		1.55	1.54
Phosphorus, g		1.31	1.23
Calcium/Phosphorus Ratio	1.2: 1		
Potassium, g		1.17	0.92
Sodium, g		0.29	0.31
Magnesium, g		0.10	0.12
Iron, mg	5.58	6.72	12.30
Copper, mg	0.41	0.36	0.77
Manganese, mg	1.00	0.17	1.17
Zinc, mg (NRC)		12.67	11.38 (NRC)
Iodine, mg	0.055	0.00	0.055
Selenium, mg		0.07	0.02

VITAMINS			
Vit A IU		2990.48	1,382.86
Vit D IU	101.00	14.53	115.55
Vit E IU	2.56	2.05	4.61
Thiamine mg	0.51	0.26	0.77
Riboflavin mg		0.70	0.62
Pantothenic Acid mg		3.65	0.77
Niacin mg		17.97	9.23
B6 (Pyridoxine) mg		1.34	0.62
Folic acid mg	0.07	0.05	0.12
Biotin mg	–	–	0.013
Vit B12 mg		0.0037	0.0031
Choline mg	142.84	225.92	368.76
Taurine g	–	–	0.31

FATS	Amount in 1 pound of this recipe	Recommended per pound NRC
LA g	6.06	0.84
ALA g	0.34	0.03
AA g	0.28	0.03
EPA + DHA combined	0.16 g (EPA .06, DHA .10)	0.015 g
Overall omega-6/omega-3 ratio: 11.75: 1		615 kcal per pound

CAT Chicken, turkey, beef, organs and veggies with bone meal + krill: NO Eggs, NO sardines

MACRONUTRIENTS	As fed	% of calories	DM
Protein	16%	49%	62%
Fat	7%	48%	27%
Moisture	74%		0%
Ash	1.8%		7%
Carbohydrate	0.8%	2%	3%

MICRONUTRIENTS	Additional nutrients needed per pound	Nutrient per pound of this recipe	AAFCO requirement per pound this recipe
Calcium, g		1.55	1.46
Phosphorus, g		1.35	1.17
Calcium/Phosphorus Ratio	1.15 : 1		
Potassium, g		1.18	0.88
Sodium, g		0.29	0.29
Magnesium, g		0.10	0.12
Iron, mg	2.64	9.09	11.72
Copper, mg		0.77	0.73
Manganese, mg	0.88	0.24	1.11
Zinc, mg (NRC)		12.70	10.84 (NRC)
Iodine, mg	0.053	0.00	0.053
Selenium, mg		0.09	0.02

VITAMINS			
Vit A IU		5857.00	1,318.00
Vit D IU	94.00	16.38	110.00
Vit E IU	2.03	2.32	4.40
Thiamine mg	0.40	0.33	0.73
Riboflavin mg		1.22	0.59
Pantothenic Acid mg		4.97	0.73
Niacin mg		18.77	8.79
B6 (Pyridoxine) mg		1.43	0.59
Folic acid mg	0.06	0.06	0.12
Biotin mg	–	–	0.013
Vit B12 mg		0.0064	0.0029
Choline mg	72.60	279.00	351.00
Taurine g	–	–	0.29

FATS	Amount in 1 pound of this recipe	Recommended per pound NRC
LA g	5.40	0.84
ALA g	0.31	0.03
AA g	0.34	0.03
EPA + DHA combined	0.14 g (EPA .06, DHA .08)	0.015 g
Overall omega-6/omega-3 ratio: 12: 1		590 kcal per pound

CAT Chicken, turkey, beef, organs, sardines and veggies with bone meal + krill: NO eggs

MACRONUTRIENTS	As fed	% of calories	DM
Protein	17%	54%	65%
Fat	6%	44%	23%
Moisture	74%		0%
Ash	1.9%		7%
Carbohydrate	0.7%	2%	3%

MICRONUTRIENTS	Additional nutrients needed per pound	Nutrient per pound of this recipe	AAFCO requirement per pound this recipe
Calcium, g		1.61	1.43
Phosphorus, g		1.30	1.15
Calcium/Phosphorus Ratio	1.25: 1		
Potassium, g		1.25	0.86
Sodium, g		0.32	0.29
Magnesium, g		0.11	0.11
Iron, mg	2.55	8.90	11.50
Copper, mg		0.80	0.72
Manganese, mg	0.79	0.29	1.09
Zinc, mg (NRC)		11.16	10.60 (NRC)
Iodine, mg	0.04	0.011	0.052
Selenium, mg		0.10	0.02

VITAMINS			
Vit A IU		5891.00	1,290.00
Vit D IU		155.5	107.69
Vit E IU	1.40	2.89	4.30
Thiamine mg	0.38	0.33	0.72
Riboflavin mg		1.21	0.57
Pantothenic Acid mg		4.82	0.72
Niacin mg		22.00	8.59
B6 (Pyridoxine) mg		1.58	0.57
Folic acid mg	0.05	0.06	0.11
Biotin mg	–	–	0.013
Vit B12 mg		0.0087	0.0029
Choline mg	57.47	286.60	344.12
Taurine g	–		0.29

FATS	Amount in 1 pound of this recipe	Recommended per pound NRC
LA g	3.62	0.84
ALA g	0.24	0.03
AA g	0.41	0.03
EPA + DHA combined	0.51 g (EPA .20, DHA .31)	0.015 g
Overall omega-6/omega-3 ratio: 5: 1		575 kcal per pound

CAT Chicken, turkey, beef, organs, eggs and veggies with bone meal + krill: NO sardines

MACRONUTRIENTS	As fed	% of calories	DM
Protein	17%	54%	65%
Fat	6%	44%	23%
Moisture	74%		0%
Ash	1.8%		7%
Carbohydrate	0.9%	3%	3%

MICRONUTRIENTS	Additional nutrients needed per pound	Nutrient per pound of this recipe	AAFCO requirement per pound this recipe
Calcium, g		1.56	1.40
Phosphorus, g		1.35	1.12
Calcium/Phosphorus Ratio	1.15: 1		
Potassium, g		1.19	0.84
Sodium, g		0.30	0.28
Magnesium, g		0.11	0.11
Iron, mg	2.94	8.30	11.24
Copper, mg		0.75	0.70
Manganese, mg	0.82	0.24	1.07
Zinc, mg (NRC)		11.00	10.40 (NRC)
Iodine, mg	0.013	0.038	0.051
Selenium, mg		0.09	0.02

VITAMINS			
Vit A IU		5985.00	1,263.00
Vit D IU	59.24	46.28	105.53
Vit E IU		6.40	4.20
Thiamine mg	0.37	0.34	0.70
Riboflavin mg		1.27	0.56
Pantothenic Acid mg		5.02	0.70
Niacin mg		21.00	8.43
B6 (Pyridoxine) mg		1.59	0.56
Folic acid mg	0.04	0.07	0.11
Biotin mg	–	–	0.013
Vit B12 mg		0.0066	0.0028
Choline mg		362.00	337.00
Taurine g	–	–	0.28

FATS	Amount in 1 pound of this recipe	Recommended per pound NRC
LA g	3.90	0.84
ALA g	0.18	0.03
AA g	0.39	0.03
EPA + DHA combined	0.16 g (EPA .06, DHA .1)	0.015 g
Overall omega-6/omega-3 ratio: 11.5: 1		560 kcal per pound

CAT 93% beef only (no organs) with veggie mix and no other additions

MACRONUTRIENTS	As fed	% of calories	DM
Protein	18%	57%	71%
Fat	6%	43%	24%
Moisture	74%		0%
Ash	1.8%		7%
Carbohydrate	0.3%	1%	1%

MICRONUTRIENTS	Additional nutrients needed per pound	Nutrient per pound of this recipe	AAFCO requirement per pound this recipe
Calcium, g	1.39	0.06	1.45
Phosphorus, g	0.39	0.77	1.16
Calcium/Phosphorus Ratio	0.08: 1		
Potassium, g		1.48	0.87
Sodium, g	0.02	0.27	0.29
Magnesium, g	0.02	0.09	0.12
Iron, mg	2.25	9.32	11.57
Copper, mg	0.40	0.32	0.72
Manganese, mg	0.95	0.15	1.10
Zinc, mg (NRC)		19.45	10.90 (NRC)
Iodine, mg	0.522	0.0522	0.0522
Selenium, mg		0.07	0.02

VITAMINS			
Vit A IU		2839.00	1,302.00
Vit D IU	93.22	15.84	108.77
Vit E IU	2.04	2.30	4.34
Thiamine mg	0.53	0.20	0.72
Riboflavin mg		0.67	0.58
Pantothenic Acid mg		2.63	0.72
Niacin mg		21.00	8.70
B6 (Pyridoxine) mg		1.59	0.58
Folic acid mg	0.07	0.04	0.12
Biotin mg	–	–	0.013
Vit B12 mg		0.0087	0.0029
Choline mg	73.00	274.00	347.00
Taurine g	–	–	0.29

FATS	Amount in 1 pound of this recipe	Recommended per pound NRC
LA g	0.87	.84 (AAFCO)
ALA g	0.15	0.03
AA g	0.15	0.03
EPA + DHA combined	0.00 g (EPA .0, DHA .0)	0.015 g
Overall omega-6/omega-3 ratio: 7: 1		580 kcal per pound

CAT Chicken only (no organs) with veggie mix and no other additions

MACRONUTRIENTS	As fed	% of calories	DM
Protein	17%	48%	65%
Fat	8%	51%	30%
Moisture	73%		0%
Ash	1.7%		6%
Carbohydrate	0.3%	1%	1%

MICRONUTRIENTS	Additional nutrients needed per pound	Nutrient per pound of this recipe	AAFCO requirement per pound this recipe
Calcium, g	1.54	0.06	1.60
Phosphorus, g	0.61	0.67	1.28
Calcium/Phosphorus Ratio	0.09: 1		
Potassium, g		1.00	0.96
Sodium, g	0.03	0.29	0.32
Magnesium, g	0.03	0.10	0.13
Iron, mg	9.13	3.68	12.81
Copper, mg	0.58	0.22	0.80
Manganese, mg	1.04	0.18	1.21
Zinc, mg	6.82	5.00	11.85 (NRC)
Iodine, mg	0.058	0.00	0.058
Selenium, mg		0.06	0.02

VITAMINS			
Vit A IU		3180.00	1,441.00
Vit D IU	82.65	37.75	120.00
Vit E IU	2.76	2.00	4.80
Thiamine mg	0.51	0.29	0.80
Riboflavin mg	0.10	0.54	0.64
Pantothenic Acid mg		3.86	0.80
Niacin mg		31.00	9.61
B6 (Pyridoxine) mg		1.59	0.64
Folic acid mg	0.10	0.03	0.13
Biotin mg	–	–	0.013
Vit B12 mg	0.0019	0.0013	0.0032
Choline mg	123.09	261.18	384.27
Taurine g	–	0.00	0.32

FATS	Amount in 1 pound of this recipe	Recommended per pound NRC
LA g	7.18	0.84
ALA g	0.30	0.03
AA g	0.24	0.03
EPA + DHA combined	0.13 g (EPA .02, DHA .11)	0.015 g
Overall omega-6/omega-3 ratio: 15: 1		640 kcal per pound

CAT Turkey only (no organs) with veggie mix and no other additions

MACRONUTRIENTS	As fed	% of calories	DM
Protein	15%	44%	59%
Fat	8%	53%	32%
Moisture	74%		0%
Ash	1.8%		7%
Carbohydrate	1.1%	3%	4%

MICRONUTRIENTS	Additional nutrients needed per pound	Nutrient per pound of this recipe	AAFCO requirement per pound this recipe
Calcium, g	1.45	0.10	1.55
Phosphorus, g	0.61	0.62	1.24
Calcium/Phosphorus Ratio	1.16: 1		
Potassium, g		1.10	0.93
Sodium, g	0.04	0.27	0.31
Magnesium, g	0.04	0.08	0.12
Iron, mg	5.52	6.85	12.37
Copper, mg	0.27	0.51	0.77
Manganese, mg	1.00	0.18	1.18
Zinc, mg (NRC)		12.12	11.45 (NRC)
Iodine, mg	0.06	0.00	0.06
Selenium, mg		0.11	0.02

VITAMINS			
Vit A IU		2838.00	1,392.00
Vit D IU	116.32	0.00	116.32
Vit E IU	4.09	0.55	4.64
Thiamine mg	0.48	0.29	0.77
Riboflavin mg		0.77	0.62
Pantothenic Acid mg		3.89	0.77
Niacin mg		10.50	9.24
B6 (Pyridoxine) mg		1.25	0.62
Folic acid mg	0.06	0.06	0.12
Biotin mg	–	–	0.013
Vit B12 mg	0.0018	0.0013	0.0031
Choline mg	217.57	153.66	371.23
Taurine g	–	–	0.31

FATS	Amount in 1 pound of this recipe	Recommended per pound NRC
LA g	9.34	0.84
ALA g	0.55	0.03
AA g	0.354	0.03
EPA + DHA combined	0.07 g (EPA .0, DHA .07)	0.015 g
Overall omega-6/omega-3 ratio: 14.5: 1		620 kcal per pound

DOG Chicken, turkey, beef, organs, eggs, sardines and veggies with bone meal + krill

MACRONUTRIENTS	As fed	% of calories	DM
Protein	14%	48%	56%
Fat	5%	41%	21%
Moisture	74%		0%
Ash	2.1%		8%
Carbohydrate	3.3%	11%	13%

MICRONUTRIENTS	Additional nutrients needed per pound	Nutrient per pound of this recipe	AAFCO requirement per pound this recipe
Calcium, g		1.74	1.56
Phosphorus g		1.29	1.24
Calcium/Phosphorus ratio:	1.35: 1		
Potassium g		1.17	0.92
Sodium g		0.50	0.46
Magnesium g		0.11	0.06
Iron mg	4.72	7.69	12.42
Copper mg		1.18	1.13
Manganese mg	0.40	0.36	0.76
Zinc mg	4.30	9.16	13.50 (NRC)
Iodine mg	0.19	0.04	0.23
Selenium mg		0.09	0.02

VITAMINS			
Vit A IU		8514.27	771.65
Vit D IU		156.00	77.22
Vit E IU	1	6.56	7.56
Thiamine mg		0.32	0.16
Riboflavin mg		1.29	0.34
Pantothenic Acid mg		4.81	1.57
Niacin mg		19.09	1.78
B6 (Pyridoxine) mg		1.45	0.16
Folic acid mg		0.08	0.03
Vit B12 mg		0.01	0.0032
Choline mg		297.00	185.00

FATS	Amount in 1 pound of this recipe	Recommended per pound NRC
LA g	3.30	1.78
ALA g	0.21	0.11
AA g	0.36	0.05
EPA + DHA combined	0.47 g (EPA .18, DHA .29)	0.07 g
Overall omega-6/omega-3 ratio: 5.1: 1		540 kcal per pound

DOG chicken, turkey, beef, organs, eggs, sardines and veggies with bone meal, krill, flax, + hemp

MACRONUTRIENTS	As fed	% of calories	DM
Protein	14%	46%	55%
Fat	6%	43%	23%
Moisture	74%		0%
Ash	2.1%		8%
Carbohydrate	3.3%	11%	13%

MICRONUTRIENTS	Additional nutrients needed per pound	Nutrient per pound of this recipe	AAFCO requirement per pound this recipe
Calcium, g		1.73	1.62
Phosphorus g		1.28	1.28
Calcium/Phosphorus ratio:	1.35: 1		
Potassium g		1.17	0.95
Sodium g		0.50	0.48
Magnesium g		0.11	0.06
Iron mg	5.12	7.71	12.84
Copper mg		1.40	1.17
Manganese mg	0.41	0.37	0.78
Zinc mg	4.86	9.09	13.96 (NRC)
Iodine mg	0.20	0.04	0.24
Selenium mg		0.09	0.02

VITAMINS			
Vit A IU		8871.54	797.73
Vit D IU		171.81	79.83
Vit E IU	0.06	7.74	7.82
Thiamine mg		0.33	0.16
Riboflavin mg		1.34	0.35
Pantothenic Acid mg		4.95	1.62
Niacin mg		19.17	1.84
B6 (Pyridoxine) mg		1.46	0.16
Folic acid mg		0.08	0.03
Vit B12 mg		0.01	0.0033
Choline mg		302.00	191.48

FATS	Amount in 1 pound of this recipe	Recommended per pound NRC
LA g	4.00	1.81
ALA g	1.00	0.11
AA g	0.37	0.05
EPA + DHA combined	0.47 g (EPA .18, DHA .29)	0.07 g
Overall omega-6/omega-3 ratio: 2.55: 1		560 kcal per pound

DOG Chicken, beef, turkey, organs, eggs, sardines and veggies with ground bone + krill

MACRONUTRIENTS	As fed	% of calories	DM
Protein	14%	51%	60%
Fat	5%	43%	22%
Moisture	74%		0%
Ash	2.1%		8%
Carbohydrate	3.3%	6%	7%

MICRONUTRIENTS	Additional nutrients needed per pound	Nutrient per pound of this recipe	AAFCO requirement per pound this recipe
Calcium, g		1.87	1.44
Phosphorus g		1.39	1.15
Calcium/Phosphorus ratio:	1.34: 1		
Potassium g		1.17	0.85
Sodium g		0.54	0.43
Magnesium g		0.17	0.05
Iron mg	3.00	7.89	11.43
Copper mg		1.21	1.05
Manganese mg	0.30	0.39	0.70
Zinc mg	1.25	11.16	12.42 (NRC)
Iodine mg	0.18	0.04	0.21
Selenium mg		0.08	0.01

VITAMINS			
Vit A IU		10600.00	710.00
Vit D IU		147.00	71.00
Vit E IU	0.65	6.31	7.00
Thiamine mg		0.30	0.14
Riboflavin mg		1.30	0.31
Pantothenic Acid mg		4.60	1.45
Niacin mg		15.36	1.65
B6 (Pyridoxine) mg		1.28	0.14
Folic acid mg		0.12	0.02
Vit B12 mg		0.014	0.0030
Choline mg		303.00	170.00

FATS	Amount in 1 pound of this recipe	Recommended per pound NRC
LA g	2.40	1.80
ALA g	0.16	0.11
AA g	0.68	0.05
EPA + DHA combined	0.48 g (EPA .18, DHA .3)	0.07 g
Overall omega-6/omega-3 ratio: 4: 1		500 kcal per pound

DOG Chicken, turkey, beef and veggies with bone meal + krill: NO eggs, NO sardines, NO organs

MACRONUTRIENTS	As fed	% of calories	DM
Protein	14%	47%	58%
Fat	7%	49%	27%
Moisture	75%		0%
Ash	2.1%		8%
Carbohydrate	1.2%	4%	5%

MICRONUTRIENTS	Additional nutrients needed per pound	Nutrient per pound of this recipe	AAFCO requirement per pound this recipe
Calcium, g		1.68	1.60
Phosphorus, g		1.30	1.27
Calcium/Phosphorus ratio:	1.3: 1		
Potassium, g		1.17	0.94
Sodium, g		0.47	0.48
Magnesium, g		0.10	0.06
Iron, mg	6.63	6.10	12.73
Copper, mg	0.83	0.33	1.16
Manganese, mg	0.54	0.24	0.78
Zinc, mg (NRC)	2.66	11.18	13.84 (NRC)
Iodine, mg	0.24	0.00	0.24
Selenium, mg		0.07	0.02

VITAMINS			
Vit A IU		5049.77	791.12
Vit D IU	67.00	12.30	79.17
Vit E IU	5.48	2.27	7.75
Thiamine mg		0.26	0.16
Riboflavin mg		0.66	0.35
Pantothenic Acid mg		3.34	1.61
Niacin mg		15.98	1.83
B6 (Pyridoxine) mg		1.25	0.16
Folic acid mg		0.06	0.03
Vit B12 mg		0.0032	0.003
Choline mg	28.00	161.22	190.00

FATS	Amount in 1 pound of this recipe	Recommended per pound NRC
LA g	5.34	1.80
ALA g	0.33	0.11
AA g	.23	0.08
EPA + DHA combined	0.13 g (EPA .05, DHA .08)	0.07 g
Overall omega-6/omega-3 ratio: 11.4: 1		550 kcal per pound

DOG Chicken, turkey, beef, organs and veggies with bone meal + krill: NO eggs, NO sardines

MACRONUTRIENTS	As fed	% of calories	DM
Protein	14%	47%	58%
Fat	6%	48%	26%
Moisture	76%		0%
Ash	2.1%		9%
Carbohydrate	1.4%	5%	6%

MICRONUTRIENTS	Additional nutrients needed per pound	Nutrient per pound of this recipe	AAFCO requirement per pound this recipe
Calcium, g		1.75	1.55
Phosphorus, g		1.38	1.23
Calcium/Phosphorus ratio: 1.27: 1			
Potassium, g		1.18	0.91
Sodium, g		0.48	0.46
Magnesium, g		0.10	0.06
Iron, mg	4.00	8.30	12.27
Copper, mg		1.43	1.12
Manganese, mg	0.43	0.32	0.75
Zinc, mg (NRC)	2.26	11.12	13.51 (NRC)
Iodine, mg	0.22	0.01	0.23
Selenium, mg		0.08	0.02

VITAMINS			
Vit A IU		9146.89	762.53
Vit D IU	58.07	18.01	76.14
Vit E IU	5.00	2.48	7.47
Thiamine mg		0.34	0.15
Riboflavin mg		1.31	0.34
Pantothenic Acid mg		5.08	1.55
Niacin mg		17.30	1.76
B6 (Pyridoxine) mg		1.42	0.15
Folic acid mg		0.07	0.03
Vit B12 mg		0.01	0.0032
Choline mg		264.00	182.63

FATS	Amount in 1 pound of this recipe	Recommended per pound NRC
LA g	4.90	1.8
ALA g	0.30	0.11
AA g	0.30	0.05
EPA + DHA combined	0.12 g (EPA .05, DHA .07)	0.07 g
Overall omega-6/omega-3 ratio: 11.7: 1		535 kcal per pound

DOG Chicken, turkey, beef, organs, sardines and veggies with bone meal + krill : NO eggs

MACRONUTRIENTS	As fed	% of calories	DM
Protein	15%	54%	62%
Fat	5%	42%	22%
Moisture	76%		0%
Ash	2.1%		9%
Carbohydrate	1.3%	5%	5%

MICRONUTRIENTS	Additional nutrients needed per pound	Nutrient per pound of this recipe	AAFCO requirement per pound this recipe
Calcium, g		1.33	1.49
Phosphorus, g		1.73	1.19
Calcium/Phosphorus ratio:	1.3: 1		
Potassium, g		1.23	0.88
Sodium, g		0.50	0.44
Magnesium, g		0.11	0.06
Iron, mg	3.67	8.22	11.87
Copper, mg		1.40	1.08
Manganese, mg	0.36	0.36	0.72
Zinc, mg (NRC)	3.35	9.80	12.94 (NRC)
Iodine, mg	0.21	0.01	0.22
Selenium, mg		0.09	0.02

VITAMINS			
Vit A IU		8803.32	737.19
Vit D IU		138.56	74.00
Vit E IU	4.20	3.00	7.22
Thiamine mg		0.33	0.15
Riboflavin mg		1.28	0.33
Pantothenic Acid mg		4.86	1.50
Niacin mg		20.12	1.70
B6 (Pyridoxine) mg		1.53	0.15
Folic acid mg		0.08	0.03
Vit B12 mg		0.01	0.0031
Choline mg		253.00	177.50

FATS	Amount in 1 pound of this recipe	Recommended per pound NRC
LA g	3.19	1.8
ALA g	0.22	0.11
AA g	0.36	0.05
EPA + DHA combined	0.44 g (EPA .18, DHA .27)	0.07 g
Overall omega-6/omega-3 ratio: 5: 1		515 kcal per pound

DOG Chicken, turkey, beef, organs, eggs and veggies with bone meal + krill: NO sardines

MACRONUTRIENTS	As fed	% of calories	DM
Protein	15%	53%	62%
Fat	5%	43%	22%
Moisture	76%		0%
Ash	2.0%		8%
Carbohydrate	1.4%	5%	6%

MICRONUTRIENTS	Additional nutrients needed per pound	Nutrient per pound of this recipe	AAFCO requirement per pound this recipe
Calcium, g		1.66	1.51
Phosphorus, g		1.28	1.20
Calcium/Phosphorus ratio:	1.3: 1		
Potassium, g		1.20	0.88
Sodium, g		0.50	0.45
Magnesium, g		0.11	0.06
Iron, mg	4.25	7.70	11.97
Copper, mg		1.36	1.09
Manganese, mg	0.37	0.35	0.73
Zinc, mg (NRC)	3.69	9.32	13.00 (NRC)
Iodine, mg	0.19	0.04	0.22
Selenium, mg		0.09	0.02

VITAMINS			
Vit A IU		8477.00	744.00
Vit D IU		151.00	74.40
Vit E IU	0.97	6.31	7.28
Thiamine mg		0.33	0.15
Riboflavin mg		1.32	0.33
Pantothenic Acid mg		4.92	1.50
Niacin mg		19.64	1.72
B6 (Pyridoxine) mg		1.49	0.15
Folic acid mg		0.08	0.03
Vit B12 mg		0.01	0.0031
Choline mg		296.74	178.47

FATS	Amount in 1 pound of this recipe	Recommended per pound NRC
LA g	3.23	1.8
ALA g	0.21	0.11
AA g	0.40	0.05
EPA + DHA combined	0.45 g (EPA .17, DHA .28)	0.07 g
Overall omega-6/omega-3 ratio: 5.15: 1		520 kcal per pound

DOG 93% Beef only (no organs) with veggie mix and no other additions

MACRONUTRIENTS	As fed	% of calories	DM
Protein	16%	55%	64%
Fat	5%	41%	21%
Moisture	75%		0%
Ash	2.1%		8%
Carbohydrate*	1.0%	3%	4%

MICRONUTRIENTS	Additional nutrients needed per pound	Nutrient per pound of this recipe	AAFCO requirement per pound this recipe
Calcium, g	1.45	0.07	1.52
Phosphorus, g	0.51	0.70	1.21
Calcium/Phosphorus ratio:	1.1: 1		
Potassium, g		1.45	0.89
Sodium, g	0.20	0.25	0.45
Magnesium, g		0.09	0.06
Iron, mg	3.64	8.40	12.05
Copper, mg	0.80	0.30	1.10
Manganese, mg	0.50	0.22	0.73
Zinc, mg (NRC)		17.14	13.10 (NRC)
Iodine, mg	0.23	0.00	0.23
Selenium, mg		0.06	0.02

VITAMINS			
Vit A IU		4961.00	748.69
Vit D IU	62.95	11.90	74.92
Vit E IU	4.84	2.49	7.33
Thiamine mg		0.20	0.15
Riboflavin mg		0.63	0.33
Pantothenic Acid mg		2.48	1.52
Niacin mg		18.76	1.73
B6 (Pyridoxine) mg		1.48	0.15
Folic acid mg		0.06	0.03
Vit B12 mg		0.01	0.0031
Choline mg		245.00	179.71

FATS	Amount in 1 pound of this recipe	Recommended per pound NRC
LA g	0.78	1.8
ALA g	0.14	0.11
AA g	0.13	0.05
EPA + DHA combined	0.06 g (EPA .04, DHA .02)	0.07 g
Overall omega-6/omega-3 ratio: 6.4: 1		520 kcal per pound

DOG Chicken only (no organs) with veggie mix and no other additions

MACRONUTRIENTS	As fed	% of calories	DM
Protein	15%	66%	73%
Fat	3%	29%	14%
Moisture	78%		0%
Ash	2.0%		9%
Carbohydrate	1.2%	5%	5%

MICRONUTRIENTS	Additional nutrients needed per pound	Nutrient per pound of this recipe	AAFCO requirement per pound this recipe
Calcium, g	1.14	0.07	1.21
Phosphorus, g	0.35	0.61	0.96
Calcium/Phosphorus ratio:	1.3: 1		
Potassium, g		1.09	0.71
Sodium, g	0.04	0.32	0.36
Magnesium, g		0.10	0.05
Iron, mg	5.55	4.03	9.59
Copper, mg	0.60	0.27	0.87
Manganese, mg	0.33	0.25	0.58
Zinc, mg (NRC)	3.68	6.74	10.43 (NRC)
Iodine, mg	0.04	0.00	0.04
Selenium, mg		0.05	0.01

VITAMINS			
Vit A IU		5182.00	596.00
Vit D IU	42.60	17.00	59.65
Vit E IU	3.00	2.80	5.84
Thiamine mg		0.32	0.12
Riboflavin mg		0.73	0.26
Pantothenic Acid mg		4.56	1.21
Niacin mg		22.17	1.38
B6 (Pyridoxine) mg		1.30	0.12
Folic acid mg		0.08	0.02
Vit B12 mg	0.0013	0.0012	0.0025
Choline mg		255.00	143.08

FATS	Amount in 1 pound of this recipe	Recommended per pound NRC
LA g	2.60	1.8
ALA g	0.12	0.08
AA g	0.40	0.05
EPA + DHA combined	0.17 g (EPA .03, DHA .14)	0.07 g
Overall omega-6/omega-3 ratio: 8: 1		420 kcal per pound

DOG Turkey only (no organs) with veggie mix and no other additions

MACRONUTRIENTS	As fed	% of calories	DM
Protein	16%	59%	69%
Fat	4%	36%	19%
Moisture	76%		0%
Ash	1.8%		8%
Carbohydrate	1.5%	5%	6%

MICRONUTRIENTS	Additional nutrients needed per pound	Nutrient per pound of this recipe	AAFCO requirement per pound this recipe
Calcium, g	1.36	0.09	1.44
Phosphorus, g	0.47	0.67	1.15
Calcium/Phosphorus ratio:	0.13: 1		
Potassium, g		1.26	0.85
Sodium, g		0.47	0.43
Magnesium, g		0.10	0.05
Iron, mg	5.97	5.51	11.49
Copper, mg	0.62	0.42	1.05
Manganese, mg	0.45	0.25	0.70
Zinc, mg (NRC)	4.06	8.39	12.49 (NRC)
Iodine, mg	0.21	0.00	0.21
Selenium, mg		0.09	0.01

VITAMINS			
Vit A IU		5004.00	711.57
Vit D IU	59.49	11.90	71.43
Vit E IU	5.78	1.21	6.97
Thiamine mg		0.30	0.14
Riboflavin mg		0.66	0.31
Pantothenic Acid mg		3.38	1.44
Niacin mg		14.72	1.64
B6 (Pyridoxine) mg		1.60	0.14
Folic acid mg		0.06	0.02
Vit B12 mg	0.0016	0.0012	0.003
Choline mg		234.00	171.00

FATS	Amount in 1 pound of this recipe	Recommended per pound NRC
LA g	4.25	1.8
ALA g	0.22	0.11
AA g	0.04	0.05
EPA + DHA combined	0.13 g (EPA .04, DHA .09)	0.07 g
Overall omega-6/omega-3 ratio: 11: 1		500 kcal per pound

APPENDIX III – BONES FOR RECREATION OR DENTAL HEALTH

As you move through the "fresh diet" process, you may want to include bony meats. Bony meats can be good for dental hygiene and they can be a way to provide bone in its natural state. Though this short book can't effectively cover the many aspects of feeding whole bone to our animals, we're including some cautions and considerations so you'll have a little information.

Raw feeders usually offer two types of bones:

- "edible bones" are non-weight-bearing poultry and other relatively soft bones which clean teeth and provide minerals to the diet

- "recreational bones" are big chunks of beef or bison bone (or other animals): long bones (usually femur bones) or portions of joints. They provide dogs with the opportunity to grind, lick and chew on them, which is enjoyable for dogs and good for cleaning their teeth, but they don't offer much in the way of nutrition except for fat. Some powerful chewers can fracture teeth on recreational bones. They are also the source of many jealousy-based dog fights. Offer them separately – this is not a pack activity in most homes. Recreational bones are full of marrow. Marrow is fatty, and can cause loose stools or even pancreatitis if too much is consumed. These are important points to consider before offering whole bone, whether they are edible, whole wings/necks or femur bones.

Check with your veterinarian about your dog's bite. If it is abnormal, chewing on bones may cause dental problems. A skewed bite can easily result in fractured teeth. This is an expensive lesson for the human and an unpleasant experience for your dog.

DOGS THAT HAVE HAD RESTORATIVE DENTAL WORK SHOULD NOT HAVE WHOLE BONES OF ANY KIND. Very expensive dental work can be destroyed in no time by a dog chewing a bone.

Some people may want to feed the bony meats in the bony meat recipes whole, or unground. This is ok if you and your dog are experienced. If your animal has not been weaned onto raw food, or if there are any digestive problems, wean onto the boneless recipes first. Then wean onto the ground bone recipes. Then, if you are inclined, offer the whole bony parts like chicken necks.

Feeding raw bone (chicken necks or wings) without other food (veggies, meat etc. may cause mild to severe constipation.

Chicken necks and wings provide good dental stimulation, but not if they are swallowed whole. Teach your animal to chew before swallowing by holding the neck or wing as they chew. A firm grip with pliers often gives you the holding power you might need! The weight bearing bones of chickens, like those found in legs, are harder than necks or wings. These bones should be smashed with a heavy mallet or hammer before feeding to *experienced, healthy dogs who have demonstrated that they do well with raw bone.* Whole birds have the proper amount of bone to meat, but few beginner pets would know how to eat them.

We do not recommend feeding weight bearing bones or whole birds to novice pets.

Turkey necks might be appropriate for some dogs, but not for others. For example, if your Labrador takes a three-pound turkey neck, crunches it twice, and swallows, this would be considered inappropriate and potentially dangerous. If he settles down and crunches slowly, that's probably ok. Turkey necks vary a lot in size, and a big one could be more than a day's food for a 50-pound dog. It takes some experience and skill to be able to balance these body parts to achieve an appropriate ratio of bony meat to muscle meat, organs, vegetables and fruits. Turkeys are older than chickens when they become "meat." They have used their legs and wings and their bones are harder and thicker. Turkey wings and legs are muscular, with hard bones. No turkey parts are appropriate for whole feeding except necks and those only in appropriate proportions for the dog that has handled raw bone in smaller amounts well. Turkey legs and wings and other parts are fine if they are ground up and used in proper proportions (i.e. if you are grinding whole birds).

A novice raw feeder doing internet research will find many websites by those who feed nothing but chicken backs or leg quarters. Writers say that they have never had a problem with this very unbalanced diet. This may be true for their dogs, but we have seen problems, especially with young, growing dogs, and we wish to spare you the experience. The chart opposite shows the nutritional balance of such a diet. There is no iodine, and almost no vitamin D, two essential nutrients. Other minerals are short from 30% – 70%. 65% of the calories come from fat, as compared to about 45% in the ancestral diet.

Chicken leg quarters with skin and bone

MACRONUTRIENTS	As fed	% of calories	DM
Protein	18%	44%	60%
Fat	12%	65%	40%
Moisture	70%		0%
Ash	4%		8%

MICRONUTRIENTS	Additional nutrients needed per pound (2 cups)	Nutrient per pound of this recipe	AAFCO requirement per pound this recipe
Calcium, g		5.40	2.20
Phosphorus, g	almost double AAFCO	3.13	1.74
Calcium/Phosphorus ratio:	all life stages amount		
Potassium, g	0.40	0.90	1.29
Sodium, g	0.30	0.36	0.65
Magnesium, g		0.10	0.08
Iron, mg	13.00	4.54	17.43
Copper, mg	1.30	0.26	1.59
Manganese, mg	0.97	0.09	1.06
Zinc, mg (NRC)	10.21	8.03	18.94 (NRC)
Iodine, mg	0.33	0.00	0.33
Selenium, mg		0.06	0.02

VITAMINS			
Vit A IU	524.00	557.93	1,082.66
Vit D IU	85.57	22.68	108.34
Vit E IU	7.60	2.99	10.61
Thiamine mg		0.30	0.22
Riboflavin mg		0.74	0.48
Pantothenic Acid mg		5.03	2.20
Niacin mg		24.65	2.50
B6 (Pyridoxine) mg		1.32	0.22
Folic acid mg		0.05	0.04
Vit B12 mg	0.0031	0.0015	0.005
Choline mg	112.67	146.97	259.87

FATS	Amount in 1 pound of this recipe	Recommended per pound NRC
LA g	10.60	2.40
ALA g	0.42	0.16
AA g	0.38	0.064
EPA + DHA combined	0.28 g (EPA .14, DHA .14)	0.10 g
Overall omega-6/omega-3 ratio: 16: 1		760 kcal per pound, 2 cups

Those who feed whole bony meats as part of their diet program must still provide a balance that approximates the ancestral diet, coming as close to the balance of a prey animal as possible.

The preceding paragraphs are provided for your information only. This book does not give you a plan for providing a fresh diet based on whole raw bones. The above short discussion is not intended to cover the topic of feeding whole bone and bone composition of the diet. More in-depth discussion can be found on our DVD, *Fresh Fast Food for Our Furry Friends*.

The sample diet card opposite is filled in so you can see our intention in using these cards.

Use the fatty acid section depending on if you give daily or less than daily.

You'll fill in either the daily line (1 cap 2x day) or fill in the days of the week with the dosage you require (i.e., "¼ t" on Monday, Wednesday, and Friday)

Use the lines below to keep your other supplements, both nutrition and medical prescriptions, in order. The small section at the bottom gives a little space for observations in condition, energy, behavior or whatever you notice.

DIET CARD SAMPLE

Mauzer   4   53   5/11
NAME   AGE   WEIGHT   DATE

2 - 1# each   2 pounds per day
MEALS PER DAY   AMOUNT OF FOOD PER MEAL/DAY

meat+veggie meals	meat, veggie+egg meals	meat, veggie+sardine or salmon meals
$1^1/_2$ C meat mix	1c+2T meat mix	$1^1/_2$C meat mix
$^1/_2$C veggie mix	$^1/_2$ C veggie mix	$^1/_2$ C veggie mix
	2 egg	1 can sardine or salmon
$^3/_4$t bone meal	$^3/_4$t bone meal	$^3/_4$t bone meal
$^1/_4$t mineral supplement	$^1/_4$t mineral supplement	$^1/_4$t mineral supplement

1 cap am daily fatty acid supplement **OR**

_____ M _____ T _____ W _____ TH _____ F _____ S _____ S

NUTRITION SUPPORT PRODUCTS AND SERVING SIZE (OILS, ENZYMES, PROBIOTICS ETC.)

krill oil – mercola adult caps

probiotic – jarrowdophilus

enzymes – now super enzymes

MEDICAL ADDITIONS (MEDICATIONS AND THERAPEUTIC ADDITIONS: GLUCOSAMINE ETC.)

glucosamine

artecin 2 - 3x day for 2 weeks- recheck 5/22 with dvm

OBSERVATIONS

NAME   AGE   WEIGHT   DATE

MEALS PER DAY   AMOUNT OF FOOD PER MEAL/DAY

meat+veggie meals	meat, veggie+egg meals	meat, veggie+sardine or salmon meals
_____ meat mix	_____ meat mix	_____ meat mix
_____ veggie mix	_____ veggie mix	_____ veggie mix
	_____ egg	_____ sardine or salmon
_____ bone meal	_____ bone meal	_____ bone meal
_____ mineral supplement	_____ mineral supplement	_____ mineral supplement

_____ daily fatty acid supplement **OR**

_____ M _____ T _____ W _____ TH _____ F _____ S _____ S

NUTRITION SUPPORT PRODUCTS AND SERVING SIZE (OILS, ENZYMES, PROBIOTICS ETC.)

_____

_____

_____

_____

_____

_____

MEDICAL ADDITIONS (MEDICATIONS AND THERAPEUTIC ADDITIONS: GLUCOSAMINE ETC.)

_____

_____

_____

_____

_____

_____

OBSERVATIONS

NAME   AGE   WEIGHT   DATE

MEALS PER DAY   AMOUNT OF FOOD PER MEAL/DAY

meat+veggie meals	meat, veggie+egg meals	meat, veggie+sardine or salmon meals
_____ meat mix	_____ meat mix	_____ meat mix
_____ veggie mix	_____ veggie mix	_____ veggie mix
	_____ egg	_____ sardine or salmon
_____ bone meal	_____ bone meal	_____ bone meal
_____ mineral supplement	_____ mineral supplement	_____ mineral supplement

_____ daily fatty acid supplement **OR**

_____ M _____ T _____ W _____ TH _____ F _____ S _____ S

NUTRITION SUPPORT PRODUCTS AND SERVING SIZE (OILS, ENZYMES, PROBIOTICS ETC.)

_____

_____

_____

_____

_____

MEDICAL ADDITIONS (MEDICATIONS AND THERAPEUTIC ADDITIONS: GLUCOSAMINE ETC.)

_____

_____

_____

_____

_____

OBSERVATIONS

NAME   AGE   WEIGHT   DATE

MEALS PER DAY   AMOUNT OF FOOD PER MEAL/DAY

meat+veggie meals	meat, veggie+egg meals	meat, veggie+sardine or salmon meals
_____ meat mix	_____ meat mix	_____ meat mix
_____ veggie mix	_____ veggie mix	_____ veggie mix
	_____ egg	_____ sardine or salmon
_____ bone meal	_____ bone meal	_____ bone meal
_____ mineral supplement	_____ mineral supplement	_____ mineral supplement

_____ daily fatty acid supplement **OR**

_____ M _____ T _____ W _____ TH _____ F _____ S _____ S

NUTRITION SUPPORT PRODUCTS AND SERVING SIZE (OILS, ENZYMES, PROBIOTICS ETC.)

_____

_____

_____

_____

_____

_____

MEDICAL ADDITIONS (MEDICATIONS AND THERAPEUTIC ADDITIONS: GLUCOSAMINE ETC.)

_____

_____

_____

_____

_____

_____

OBSERVATIONS

NAME   AGE   WEIGHT   DATE

MEALS PER DAY   AMOUNT OF FOOD PER MEAL/DAY

meat+veggie meals	**meat, veggie+egg meals**	**meat, veggie+sardine or salmon meals**
_____ meat mix	_____ meat mix	_____ meat mix
_____ veggie mix	_____ veggie mix	_____ veggie mix
	_____ egg	_____ sardine or salmon
_____ bone meal	_____ bone meal	_____ bone meal
_____ mineral supplement	_____ mineral supplement	_____ mineral supplement

_____ daily fatty acid supplement **OR**

_____ M _____ T _____ W _____ TH _____ F _____ S _____ S

NUTRITION SUPPORT PRODUCTS AND SERVING SIZE (OILS, ENZYMES, PROBIOTICS ETC.)

_____

_____

_____

_____

_____

_____

MEDICAL ADDITIONS (MEDICATIONS AND THERAPEUTIC ADDITIONS: GLUCOSAMINE ETC.)

_____

_____

_____

_____

_____

_____

OBSERVATIONS

Beth has been involved in health, training, and wellness for animals and people all her adult life. In 1994 she began teaching dog training and producing education seminars on dog training and nutrition. She continues to educate herself on these topics but her focus has sharpened to animal diet and massage techniques for animals and people. Researching fresh food diets for dogs led to her work with Steve's Real Food for Pets from 1998 to 2005, during which time she taught retailers and veterinarians how to use fresh food diets and provided support for them nationwide. This work led to the writing and publication of See Spot Live Longer with Steve Brown in 2005. Seminars produced with Karen Becker led to the book you are holding, now in its 4th edition. Beth is a Licensed Massage Therapist with extensive bodywork training for animals, and is currently putting those skills to work in a swim facility for canines.

Karen Becker is a veterinarian, animal acupuncturist and homeopath practicing in Illinois. Natural Pet Animal Hospital focuses on integrative pet care for dogs, cats, birds and exotic animals. She also runs Covenant Wildlife Rehabilitation, a non-profit facility that cares for injured and orphaned Chicago area wildlife. She is the chief veterinarian for mercolahealthypets.com.

Together, for the past ten years, they have been producing seminars, DVDs and books to help people take charge of their dog's and cat's health.

Our thanks and appreciation to Steve Brown, creator of Steve's Real Food and many other innovative products for dogs, for his work on analysis and food composition which helped us give you these recipes.

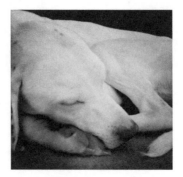